I0480619

This book belongs to

_____

_____

_____

COMPLETE SKELETON OF A HORSE

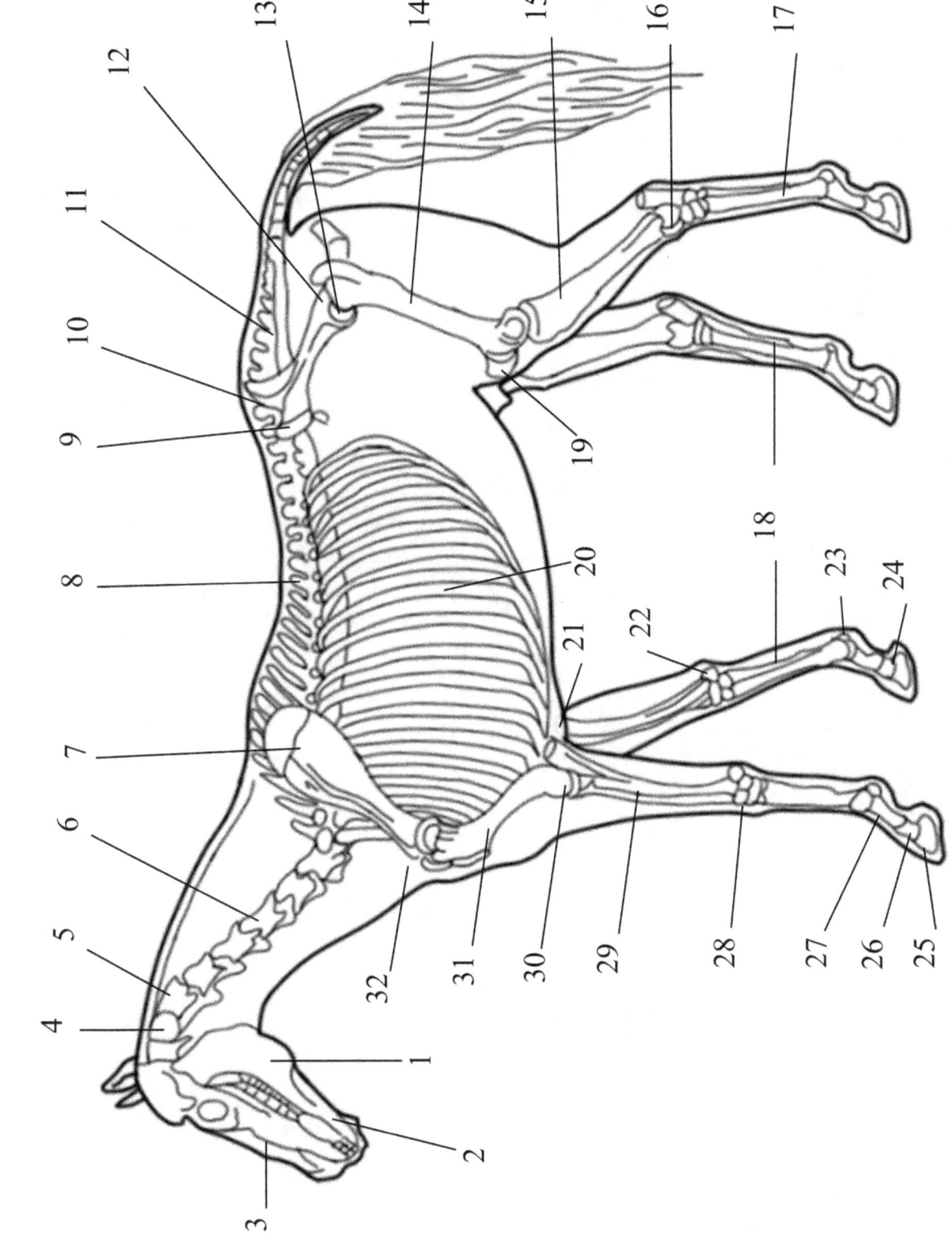

FORELIMB

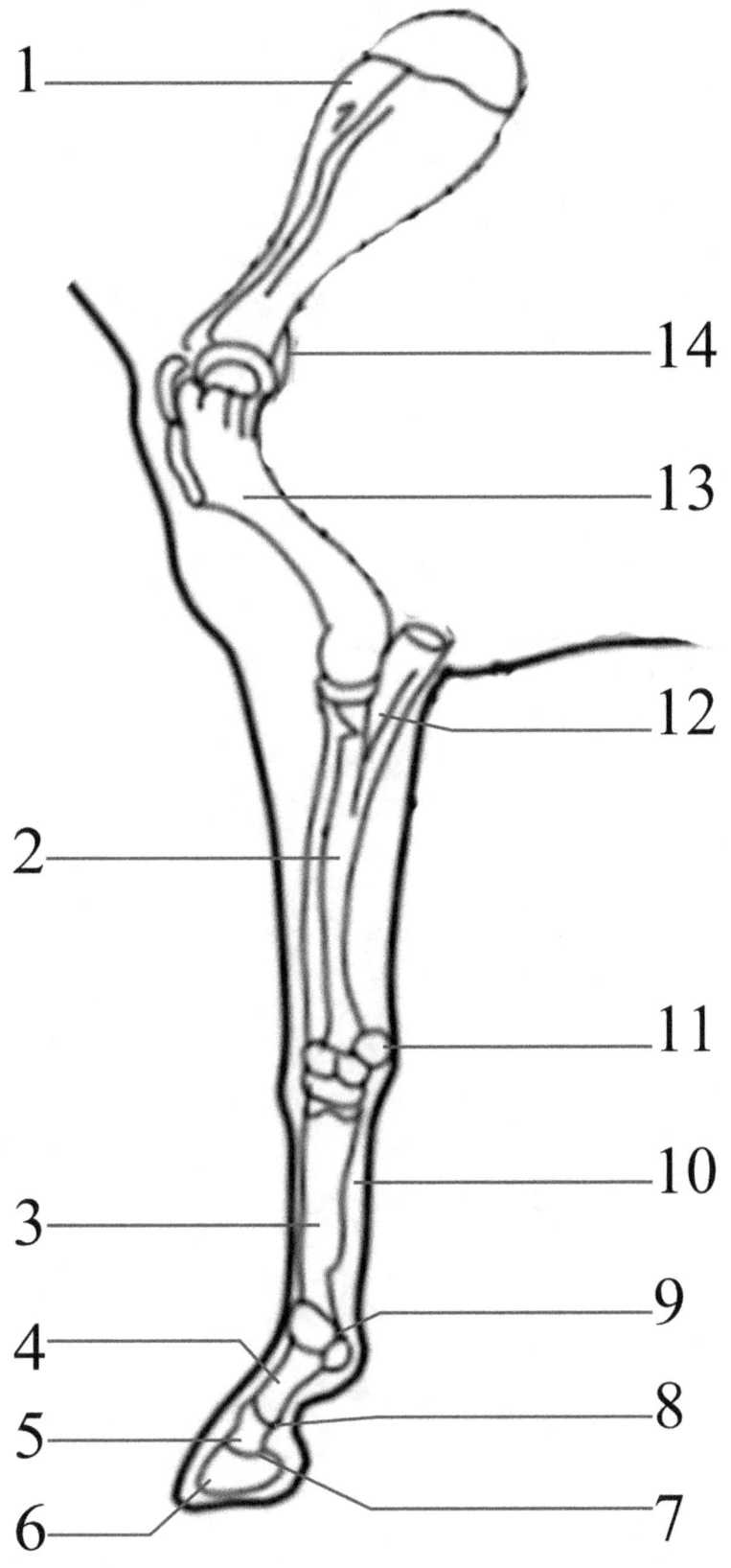

1
14
13
12
2
11
10
3
9
4
8
5
7
6

ANTERIOR VIEW OF EQUINE CARPUS

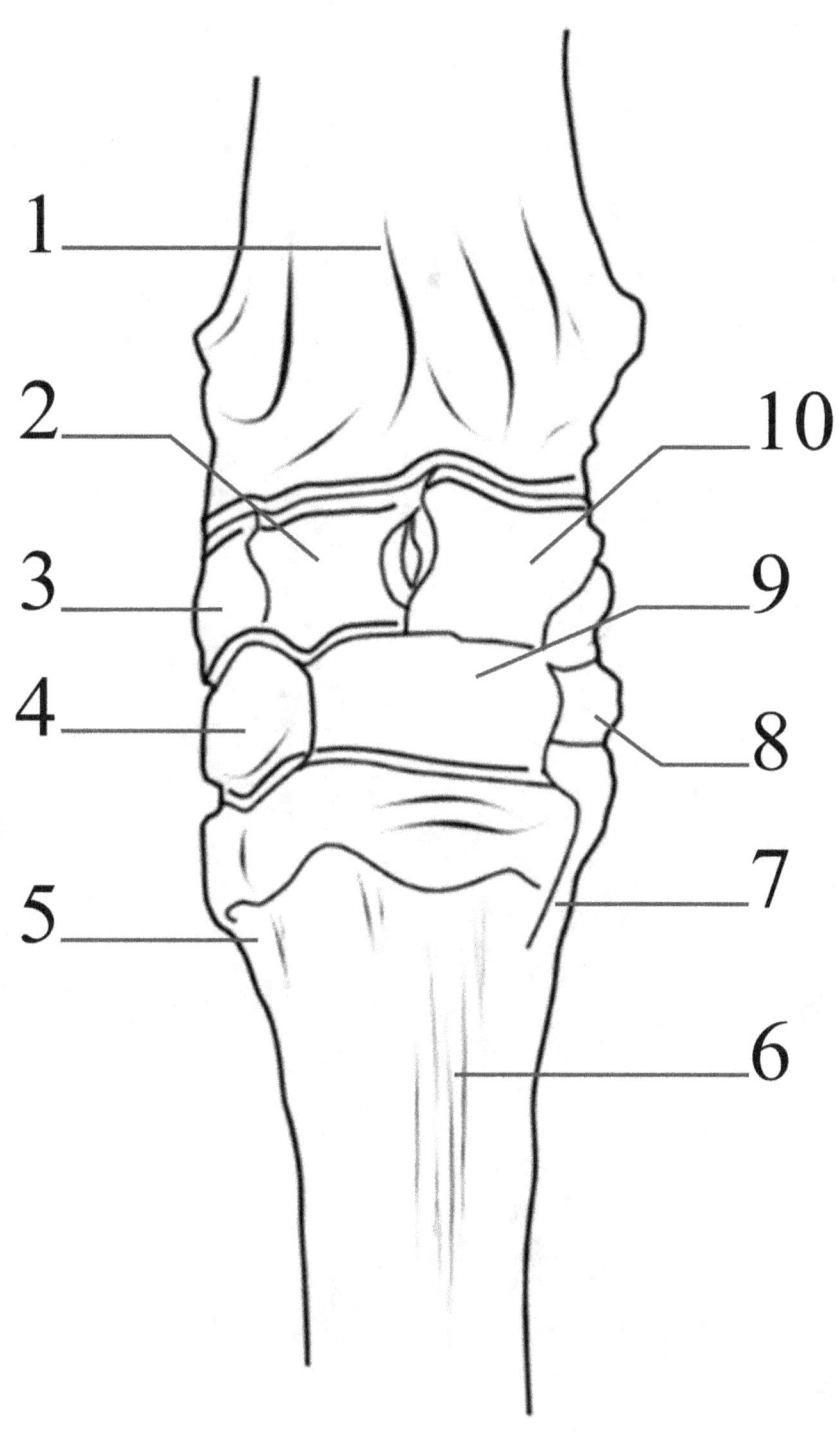

HIND LIMB

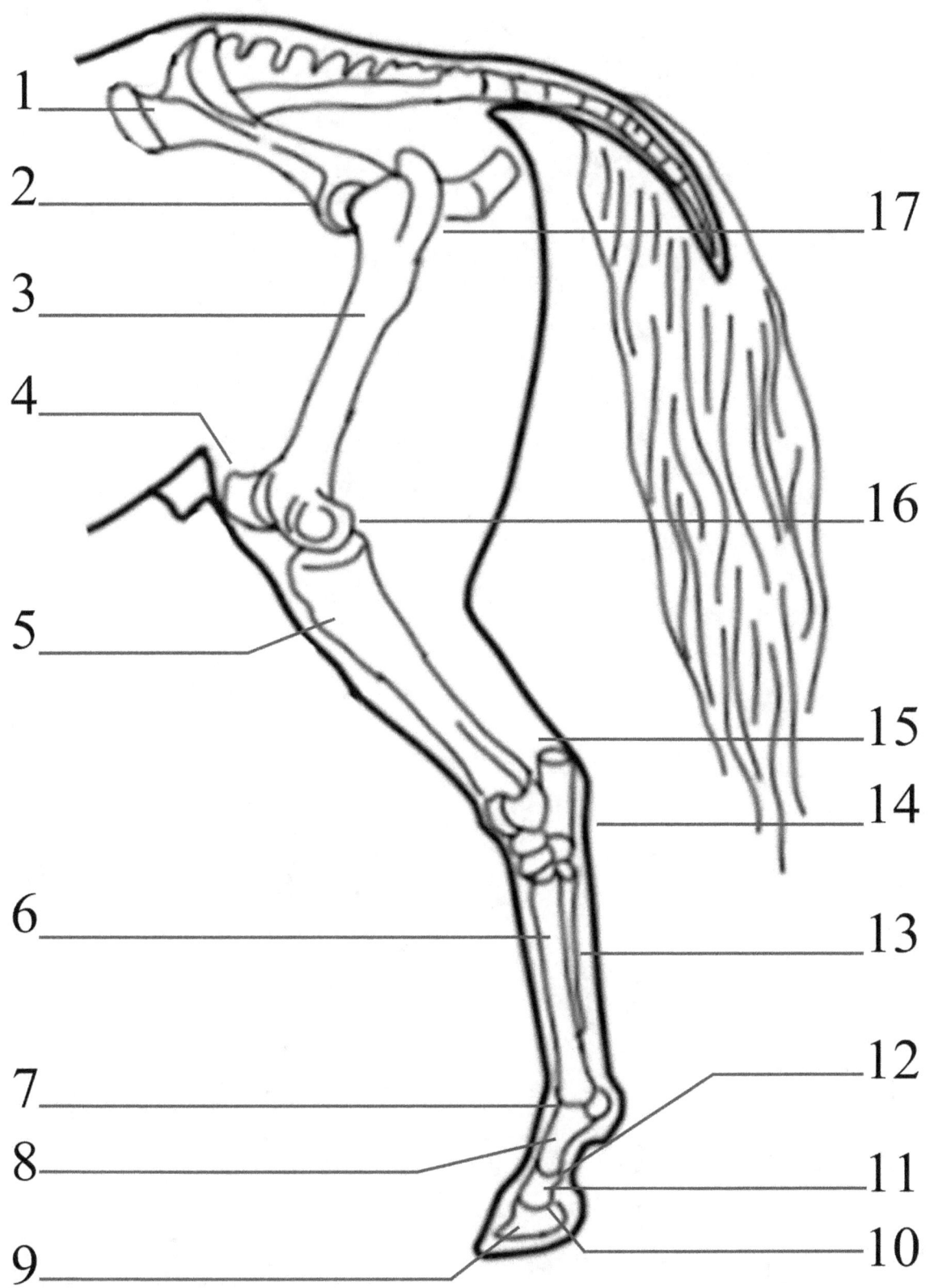

EQUINE TARSUS AND STIFLE

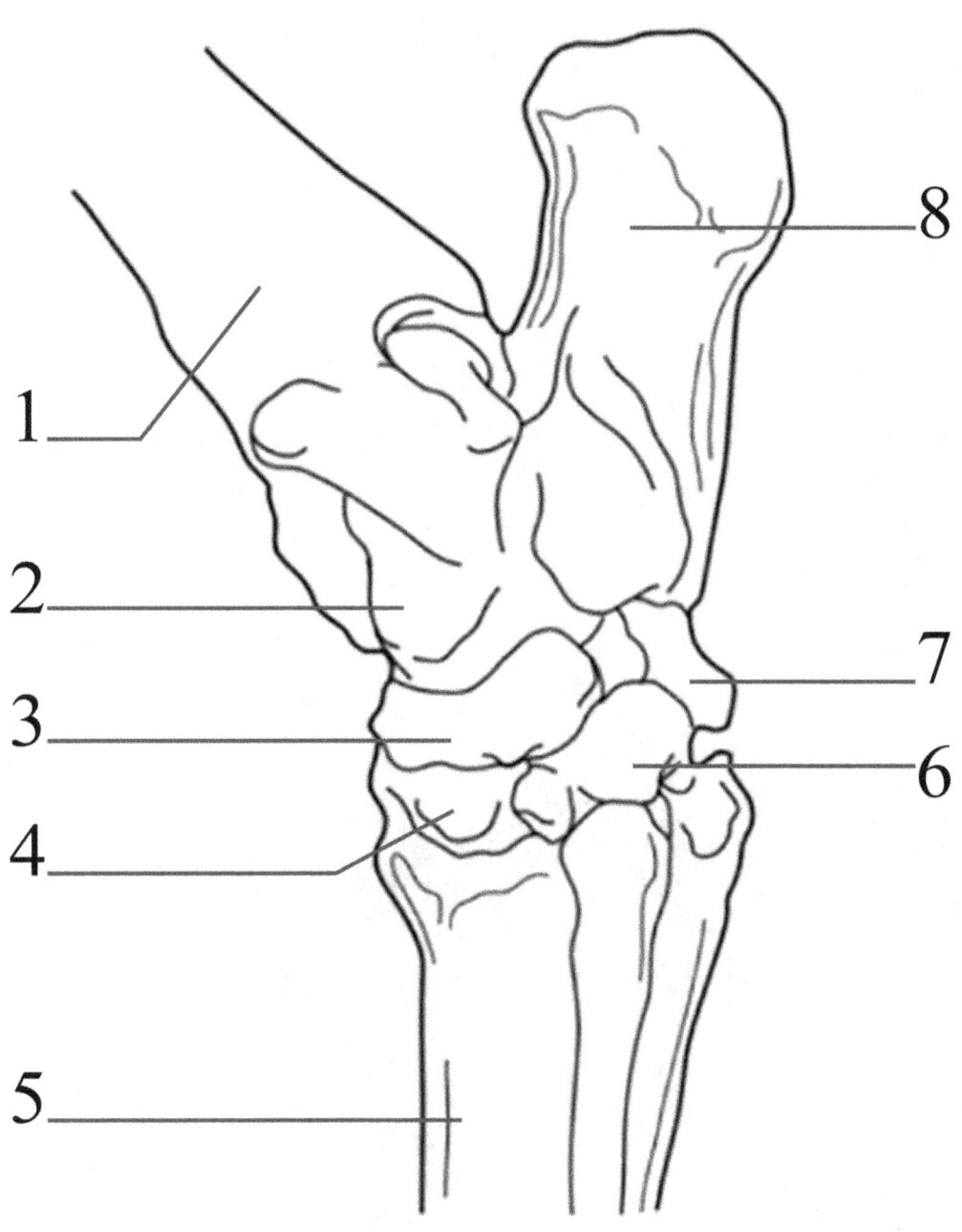

1

2

3

4

5

6

7

8

SPINAL CORD OF A YOUNG HORSE

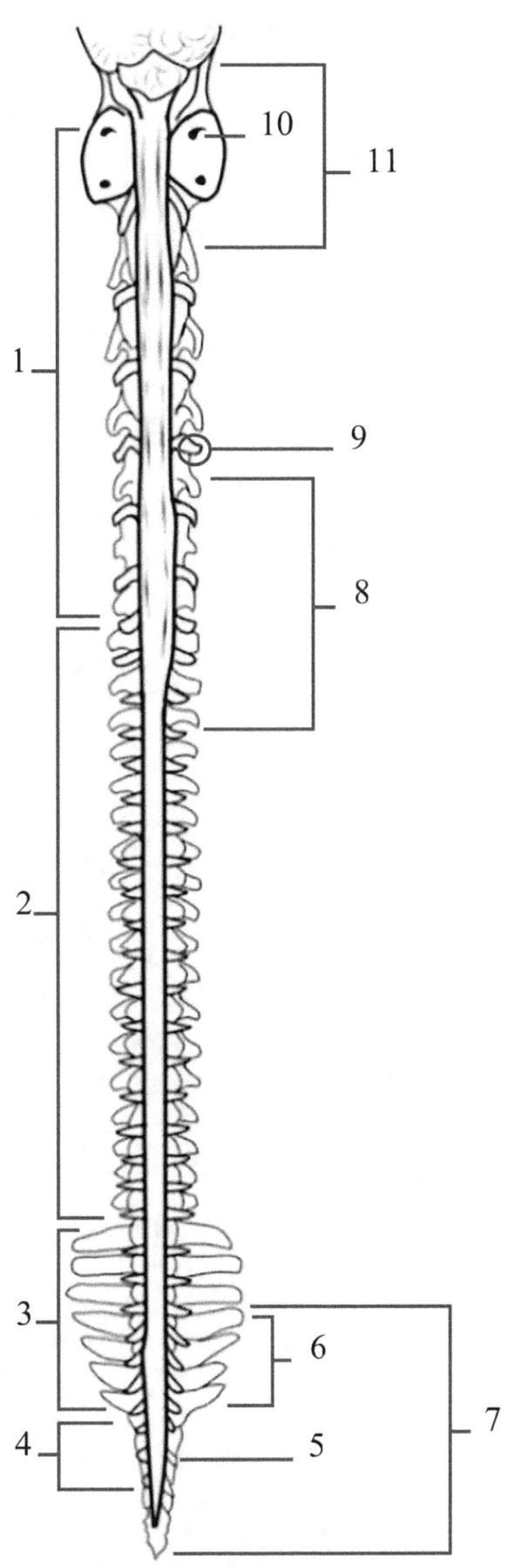

HORSE SKULL

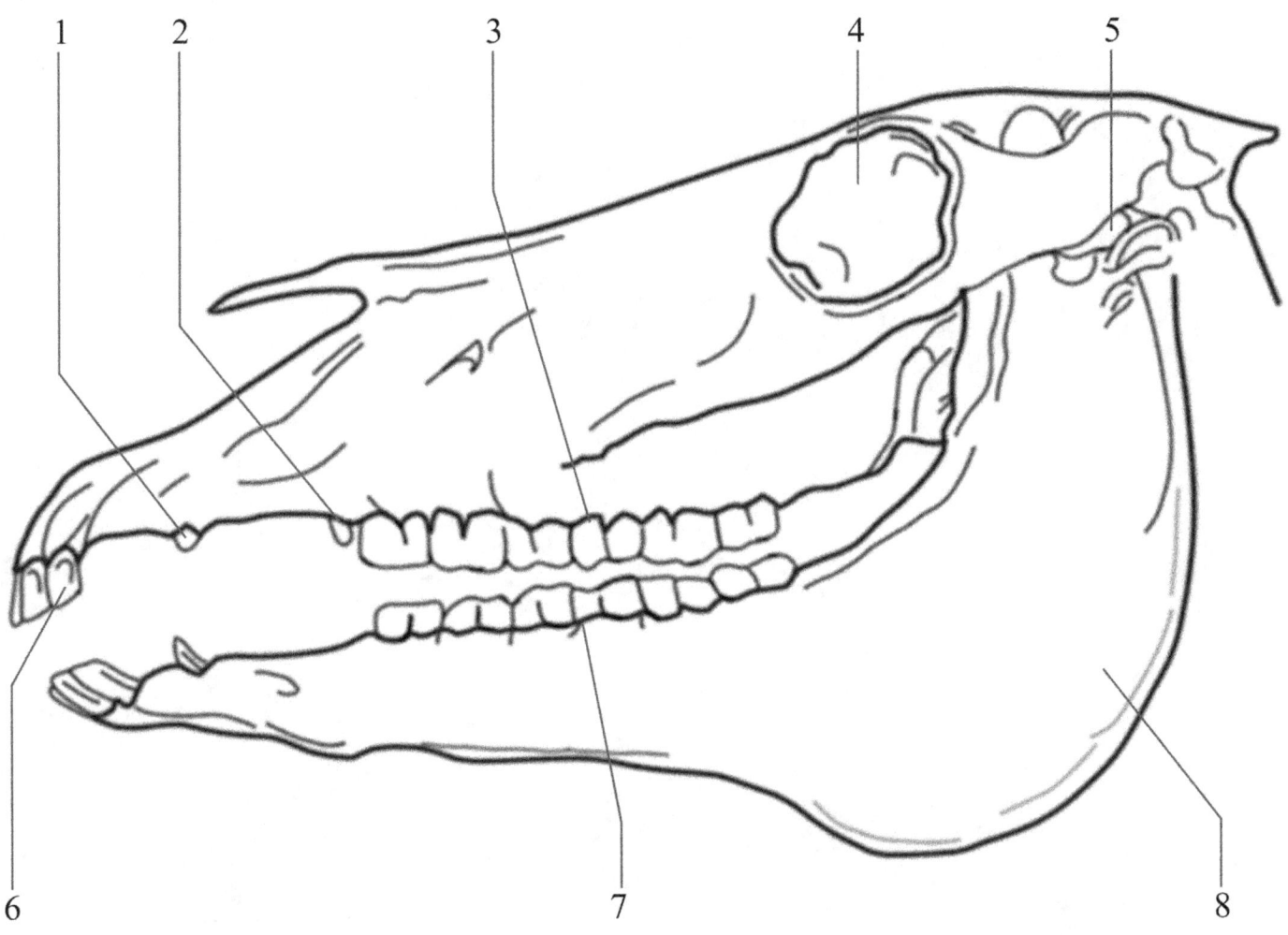

EQUINE DENTISTRY

Maxilla (Upper)   Mandible (Lower)

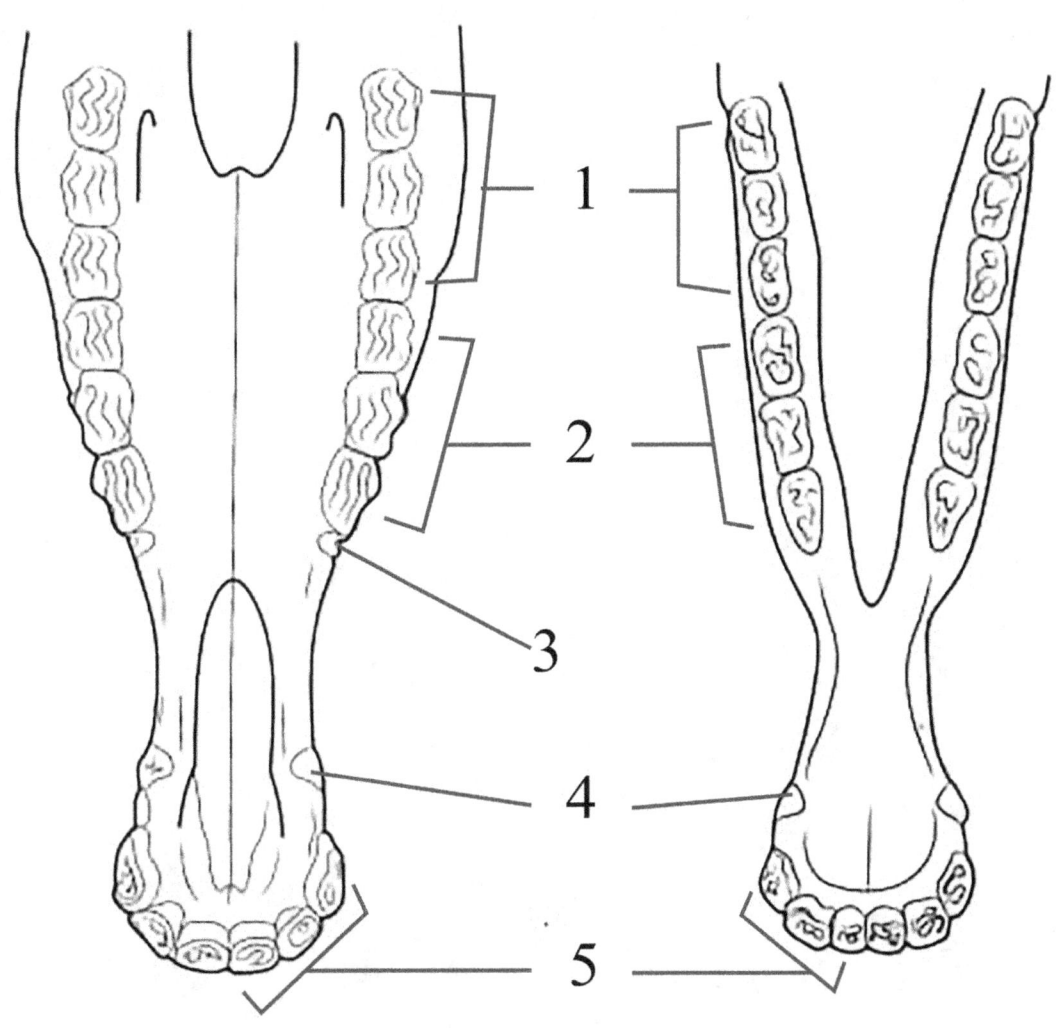

HORSE HOOF

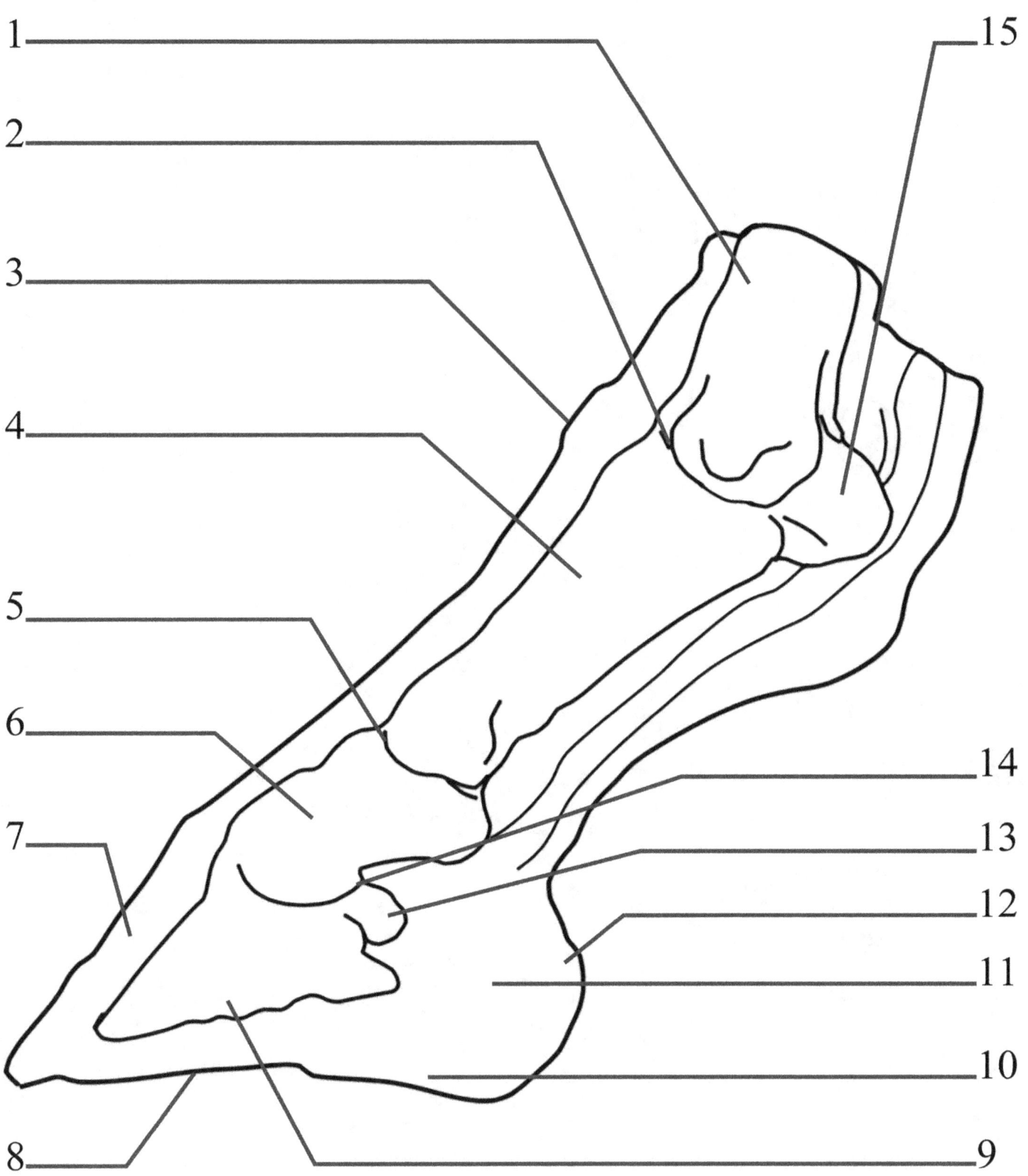

1
2
3
4
5
6
7
8

15
14
13
12
11
10
9

EXTERIOR VIEW AND GROUND SURFACE OF HORSE HOOF

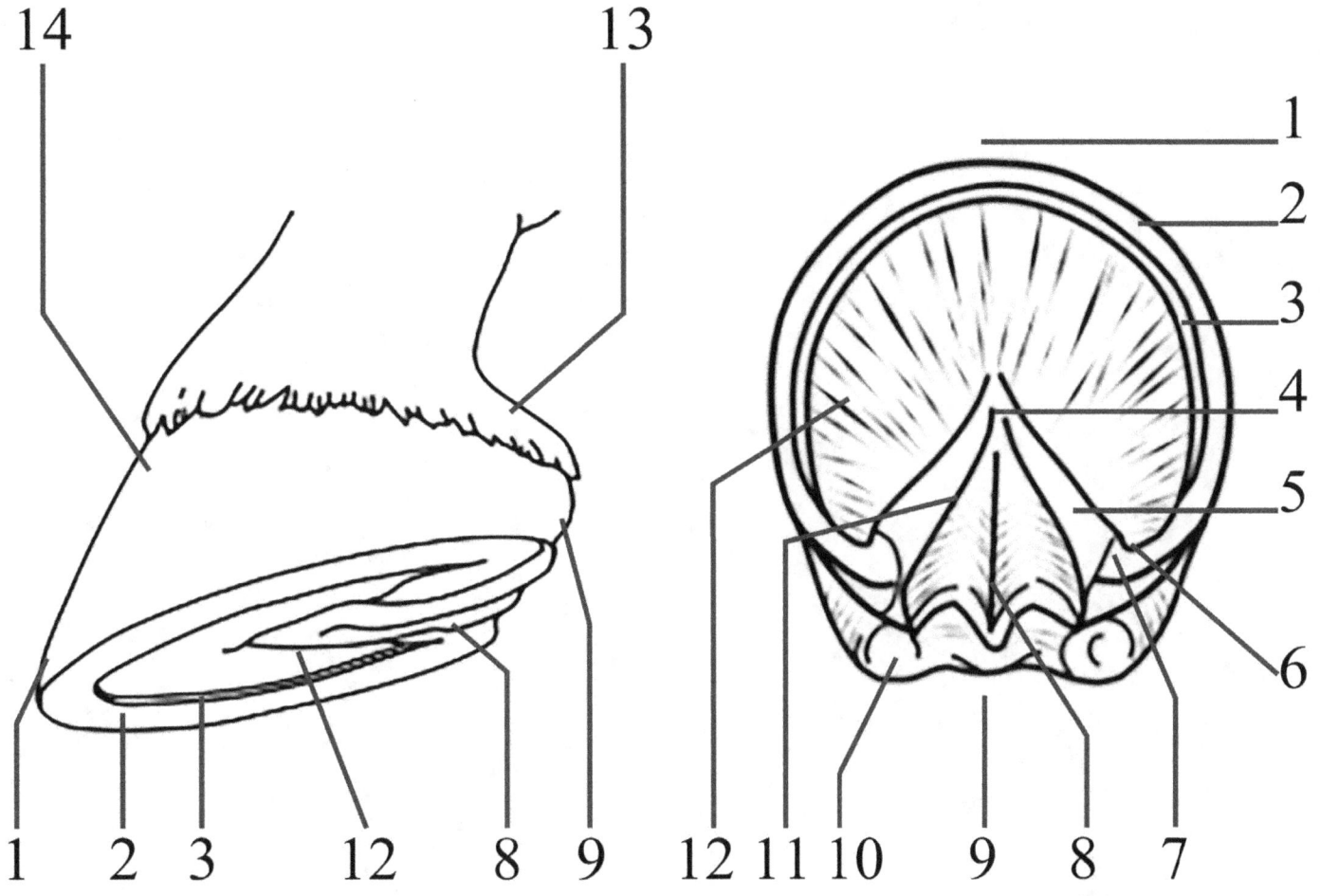

LIMB TENDON AND LIGAMENT

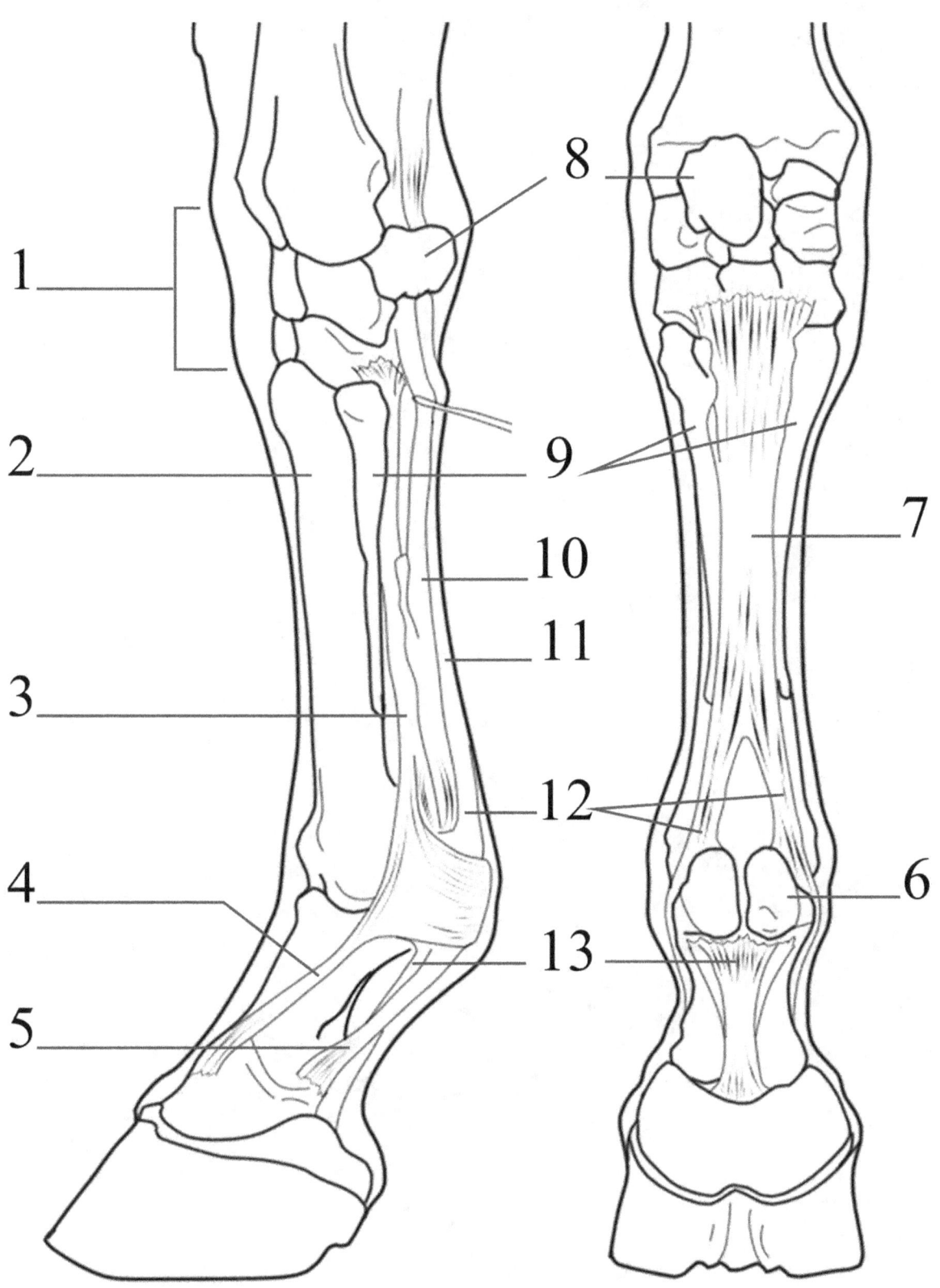

DORSAL VIEW OF HORSE BRAIN WITH SECTIONED LEFT HEMISPHERE

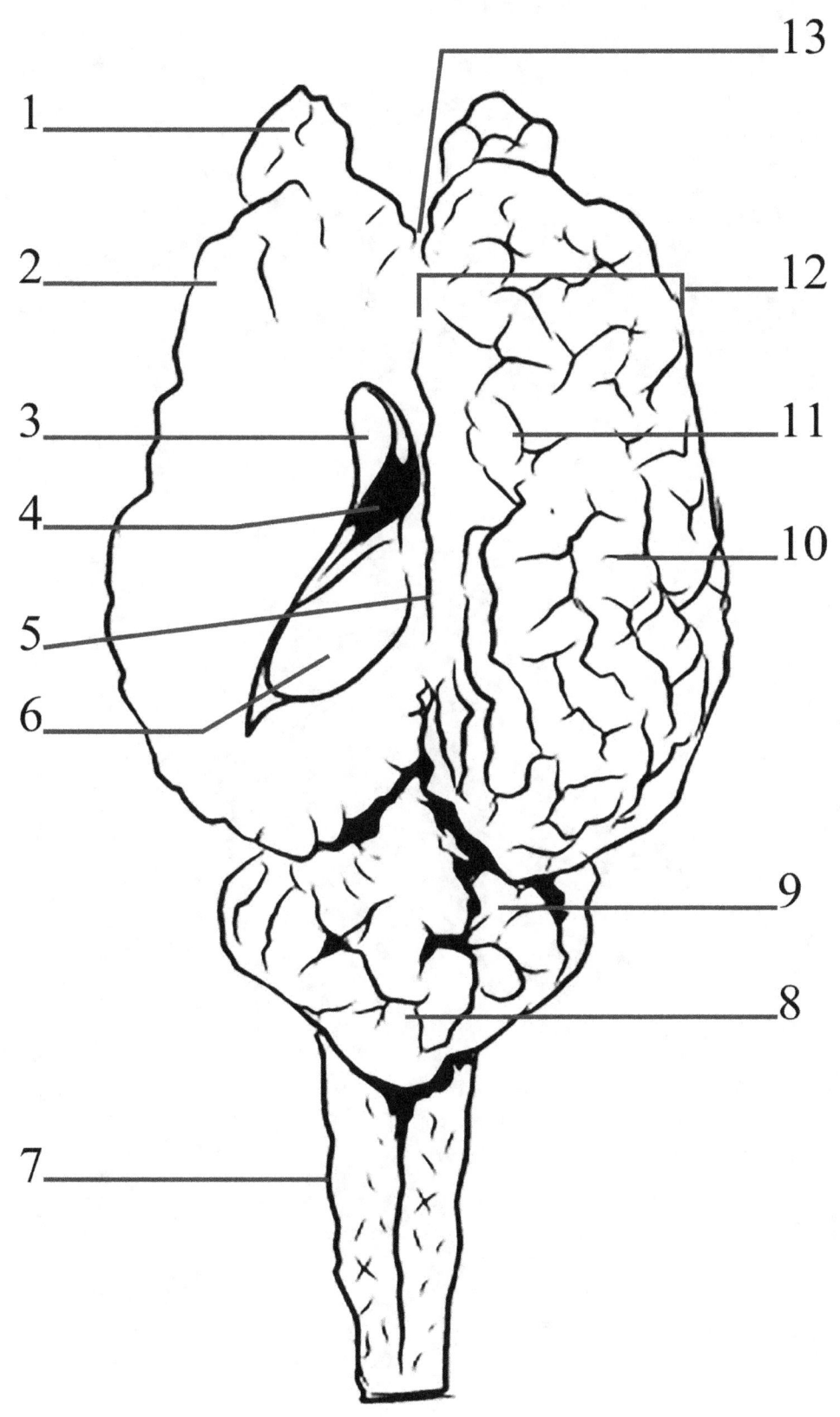

EQUINE EYE

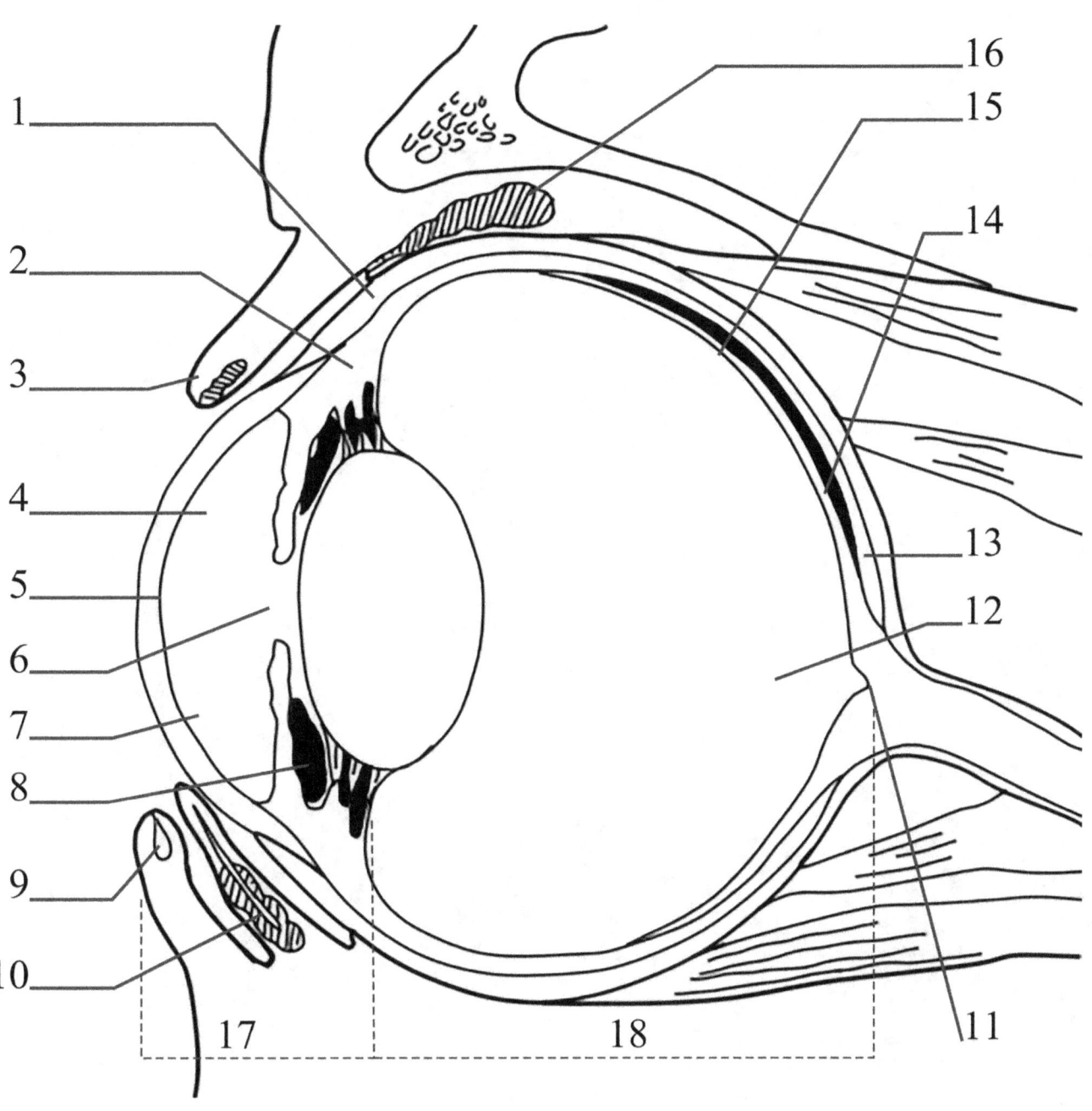

EXTERIOR VIEW OF EQUINE EYE

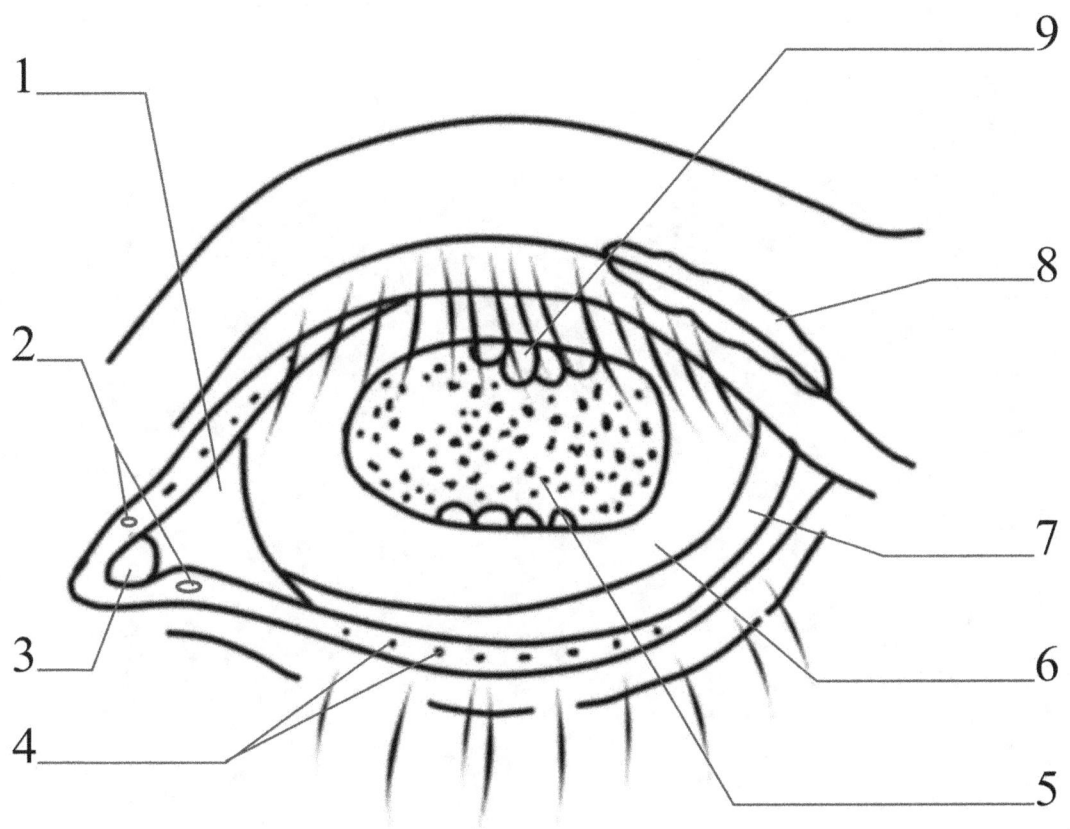

ANATOMY OF A HORSE TONGUE

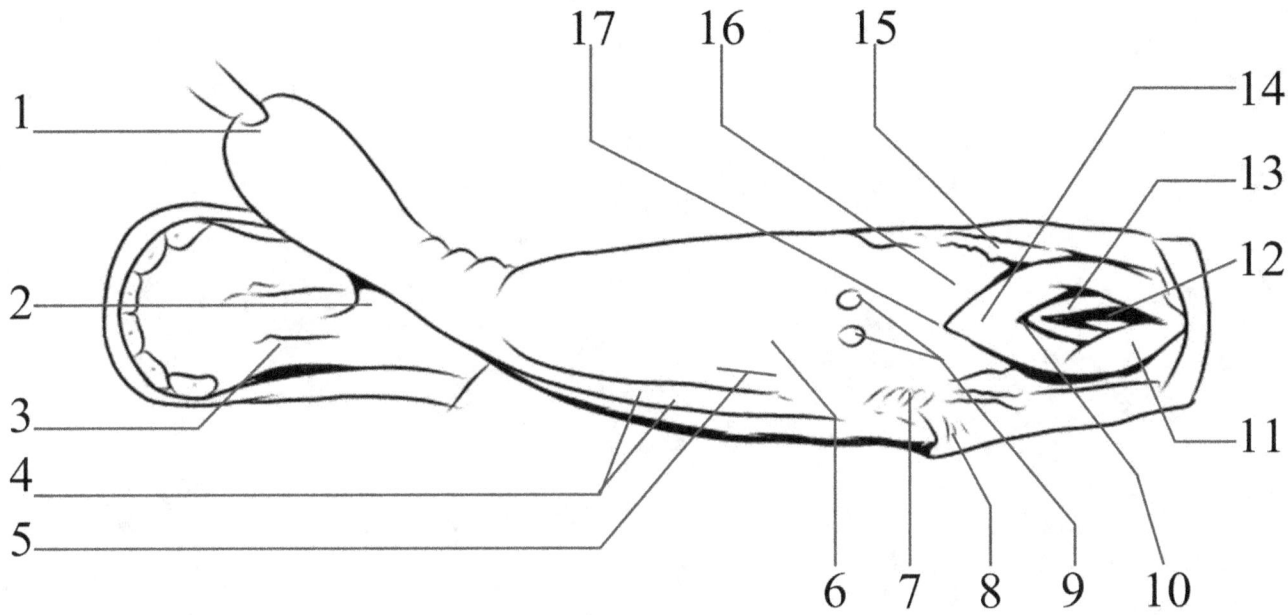

EQUINE EAR

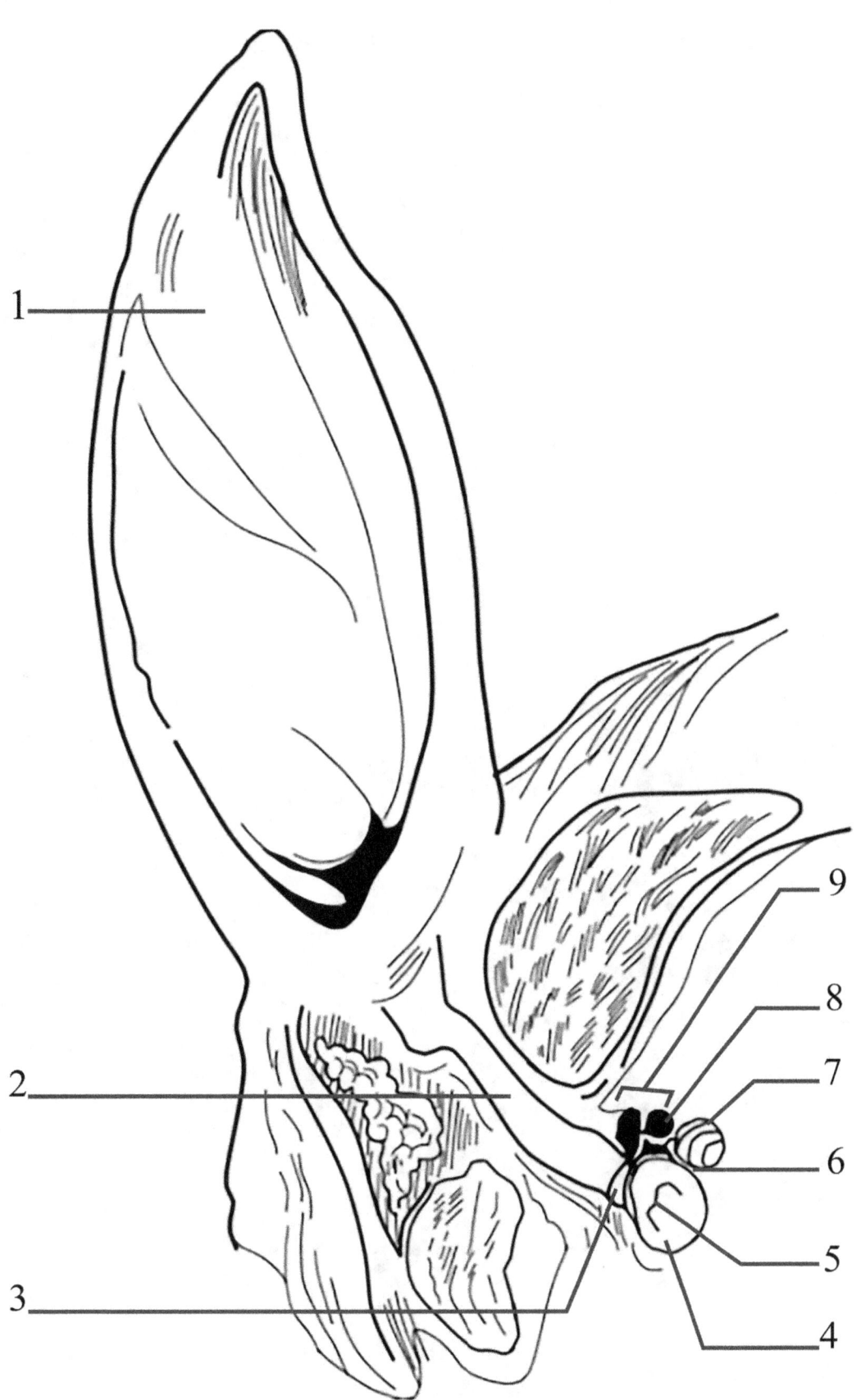

STRUCTURE OF HORSE SKIN

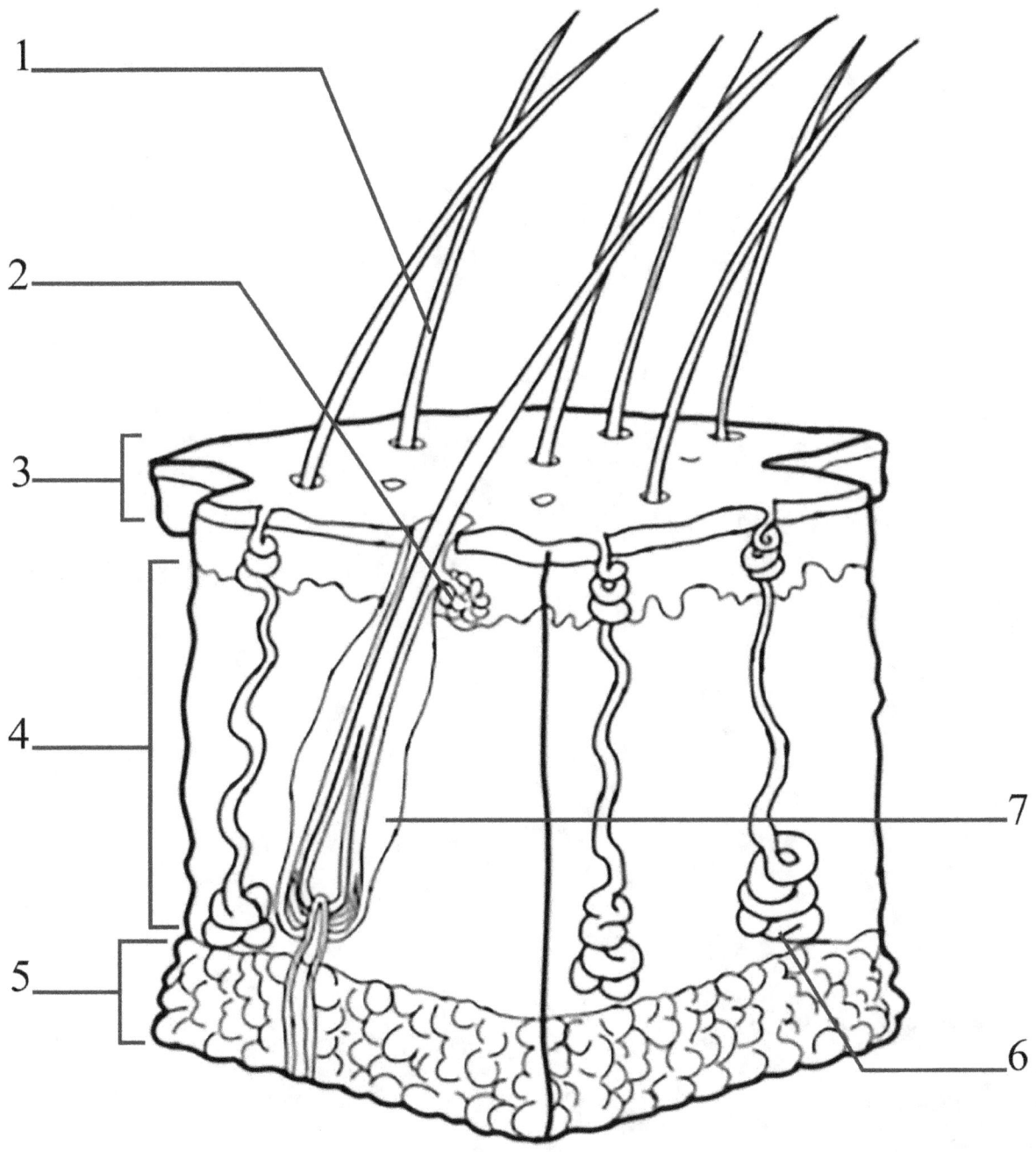

1

2

3

4

5

7

6

EQUINE RESPIRATORY SYSTEM

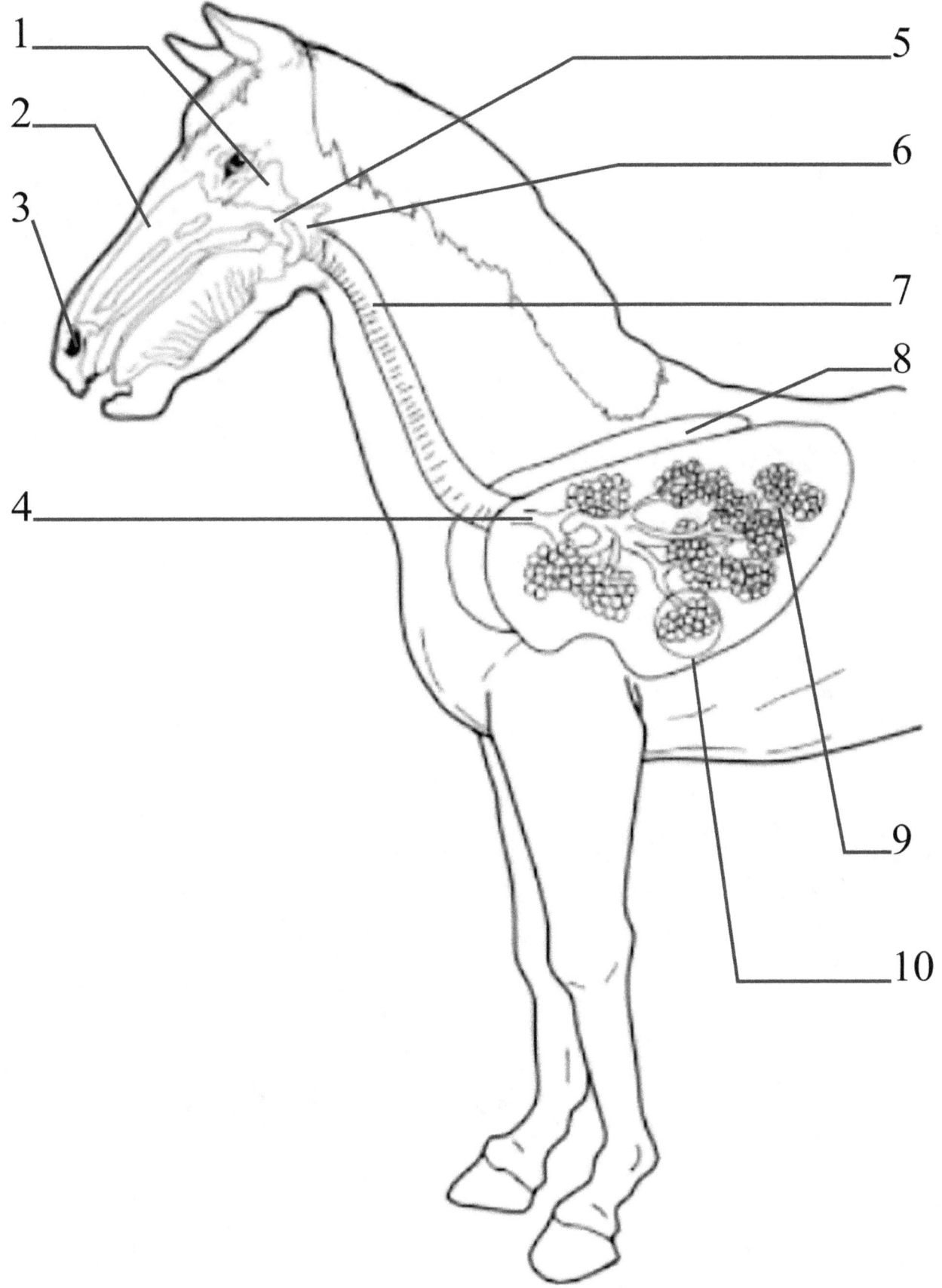

VENTRAL VIEW OF THE LUNGS

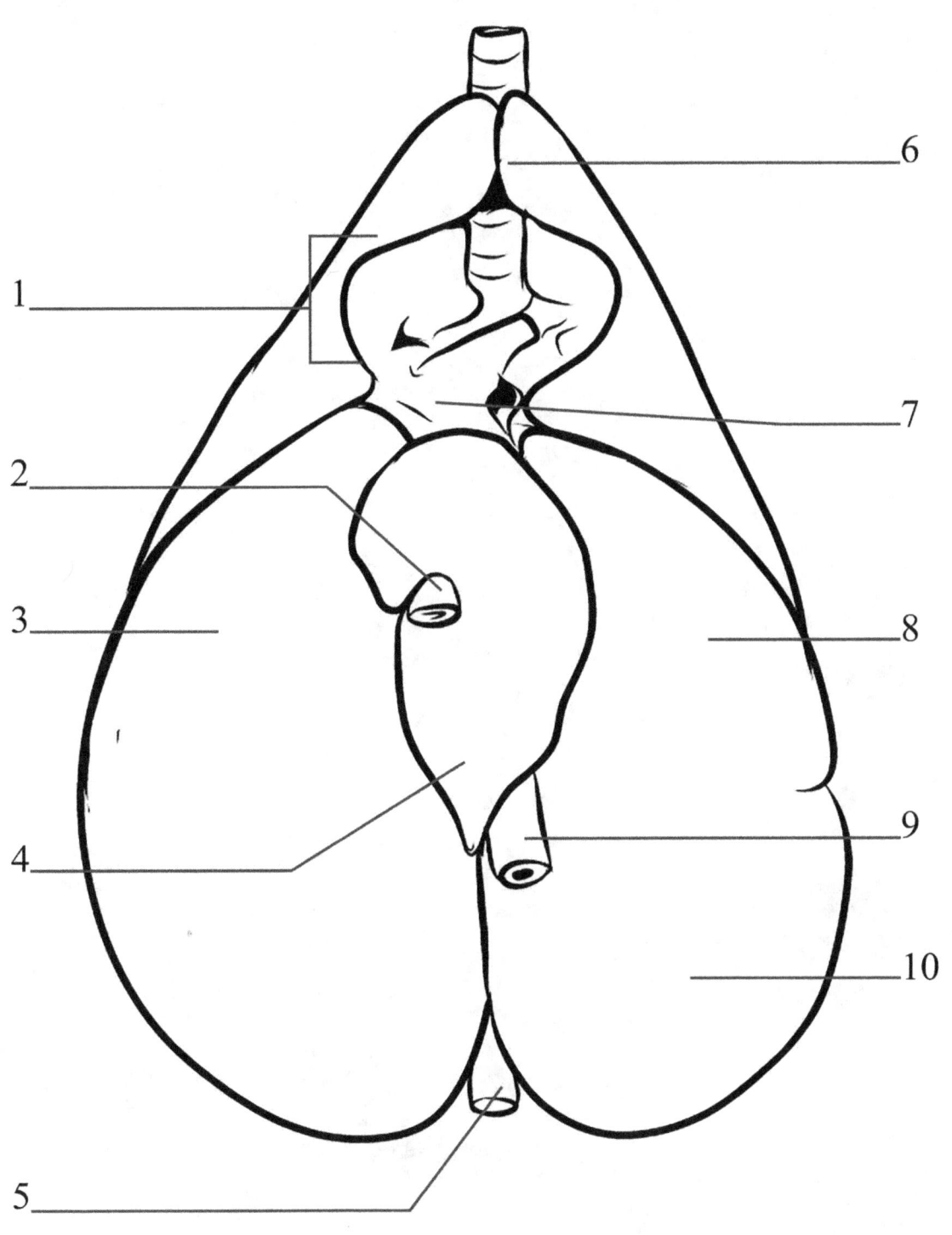

1

2

3

4

5

6

7

8

9

10

DORSAL VIEW OF BRONCHIAL TREE

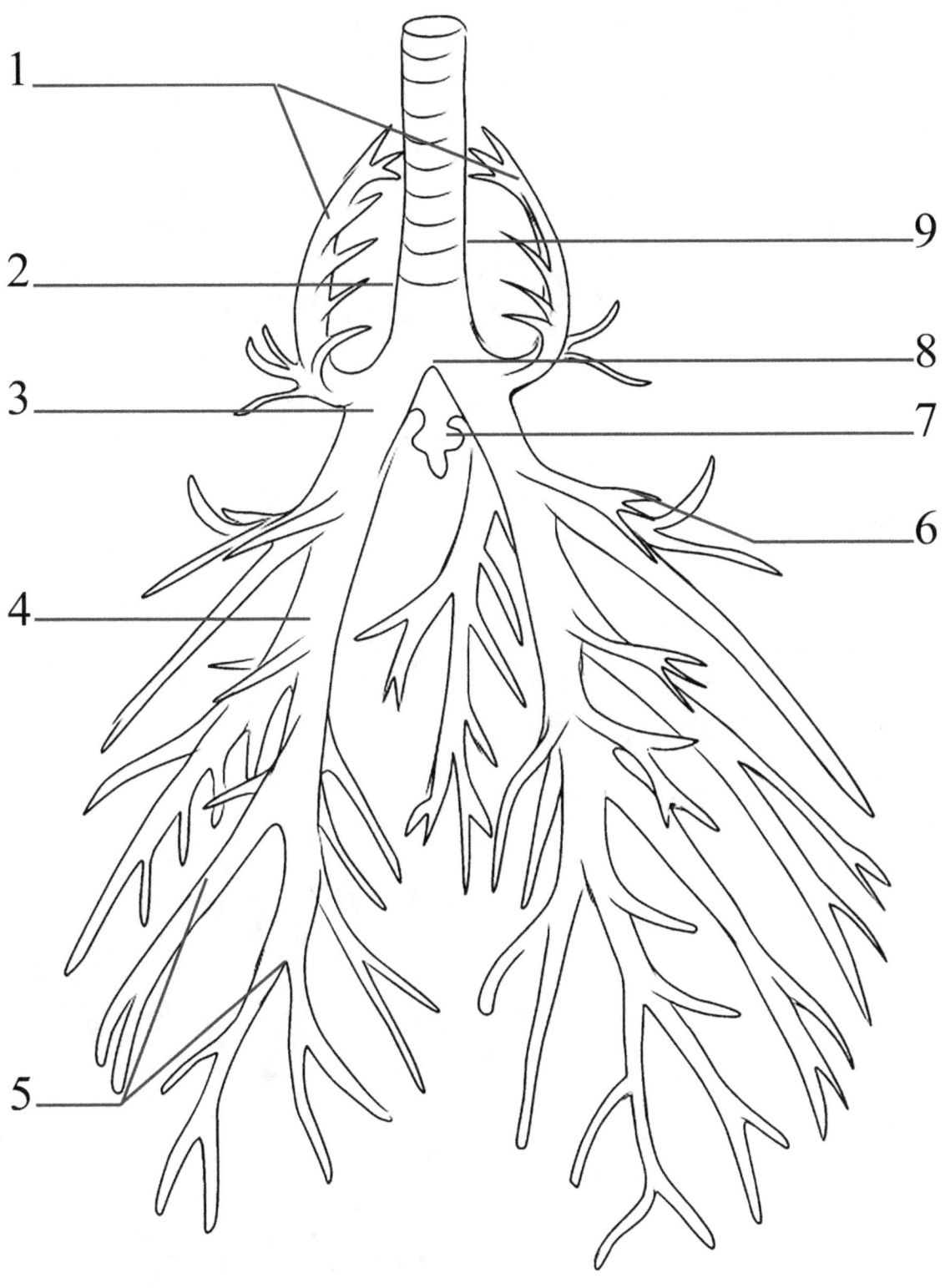

DIGESTIVE SYSTEM OF A HORSE

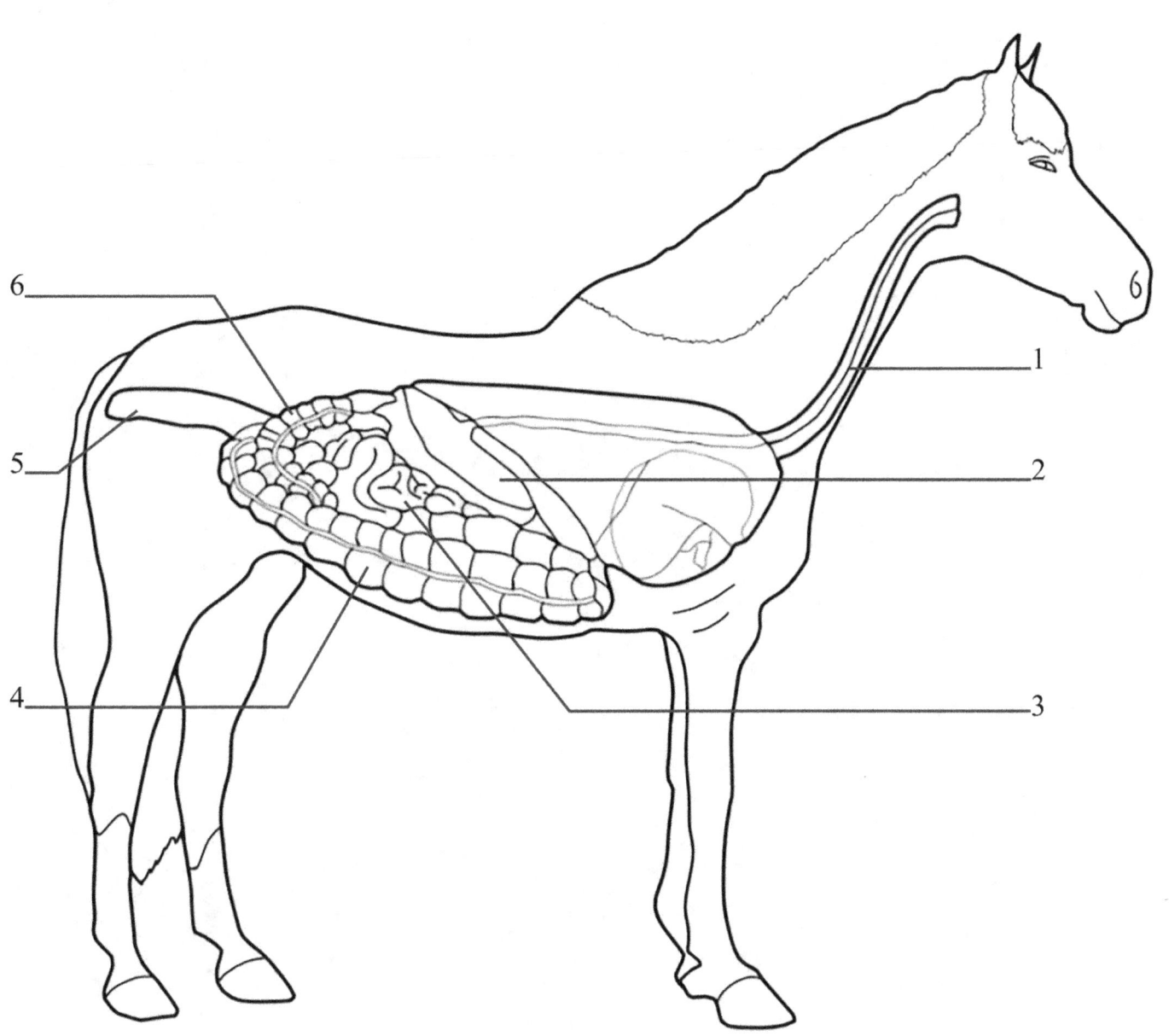

THE EQUINE STOMACH

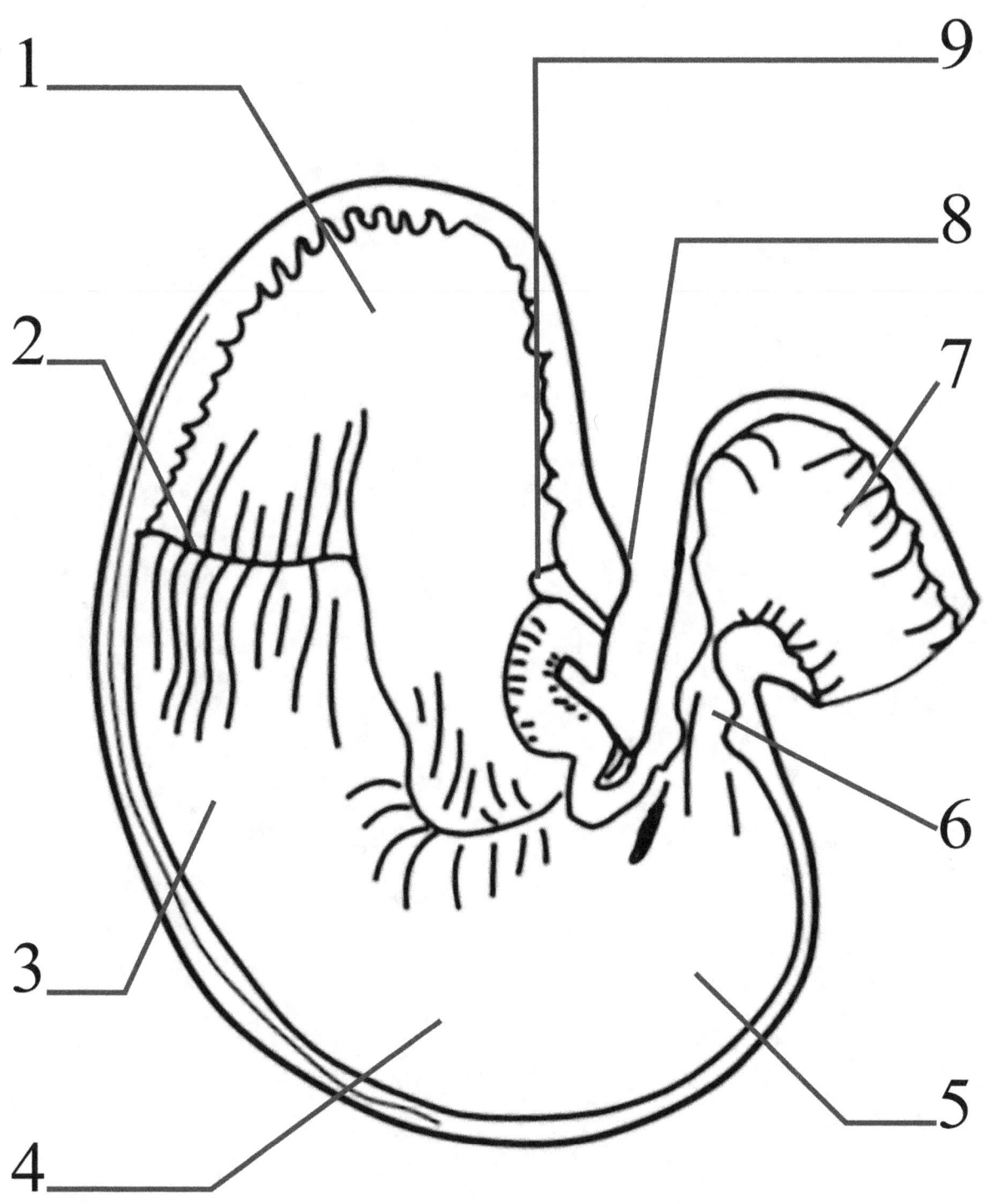

LARGE INTESTINE OF A HORSE

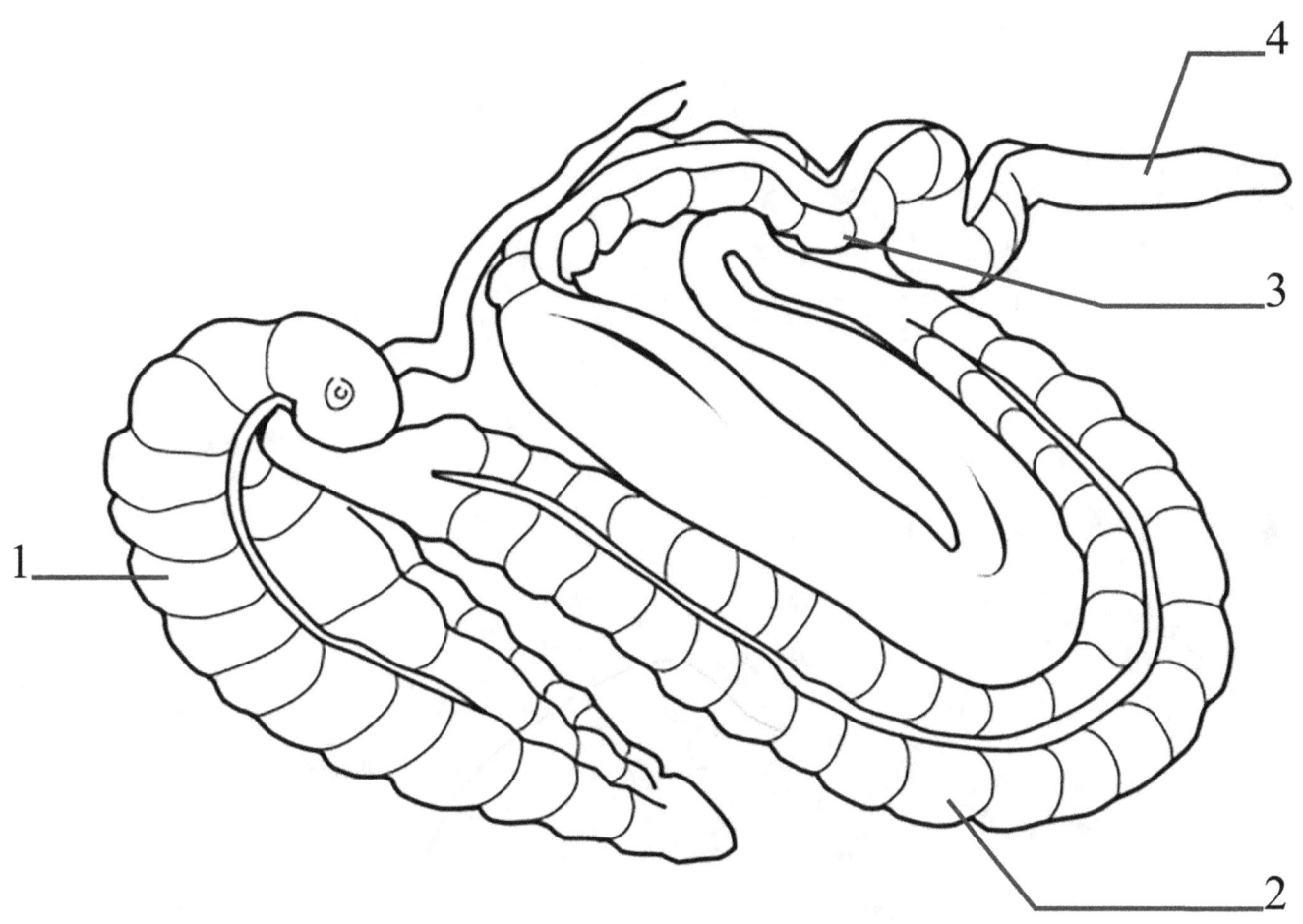

EQUINE HEART

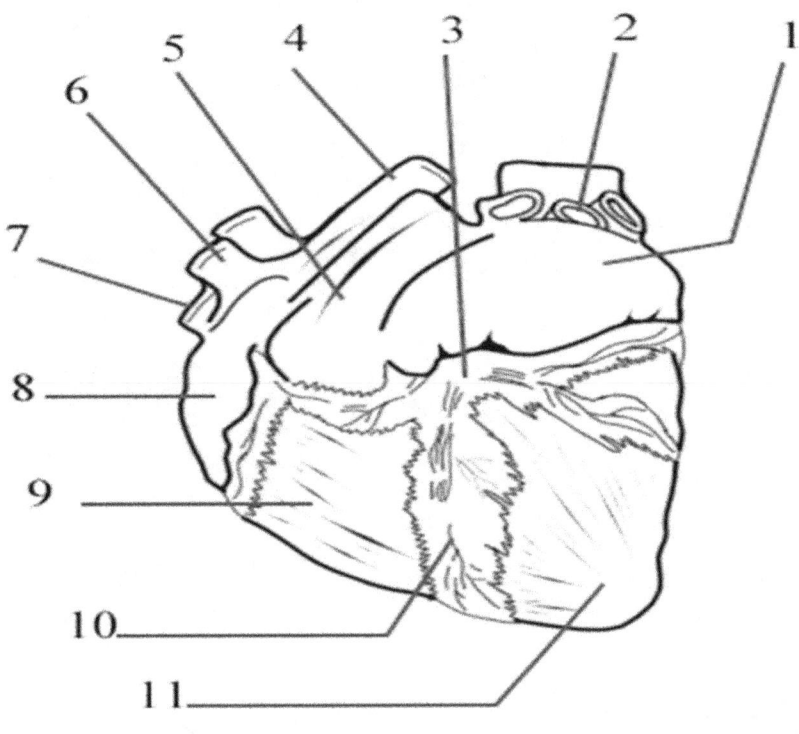

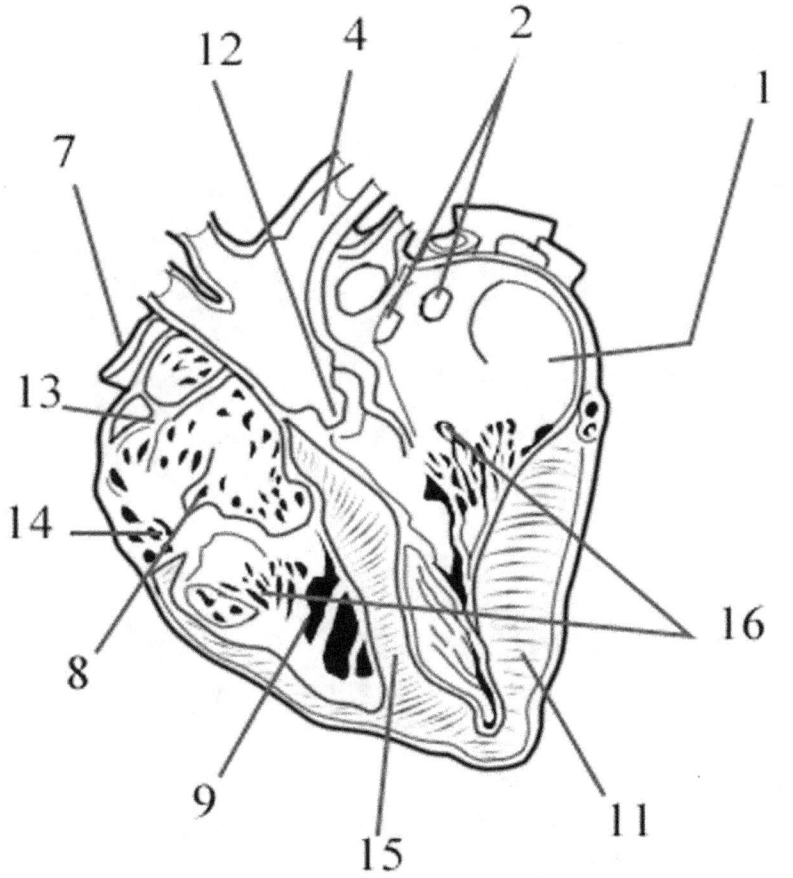

STALLION URINARY SYSTEM

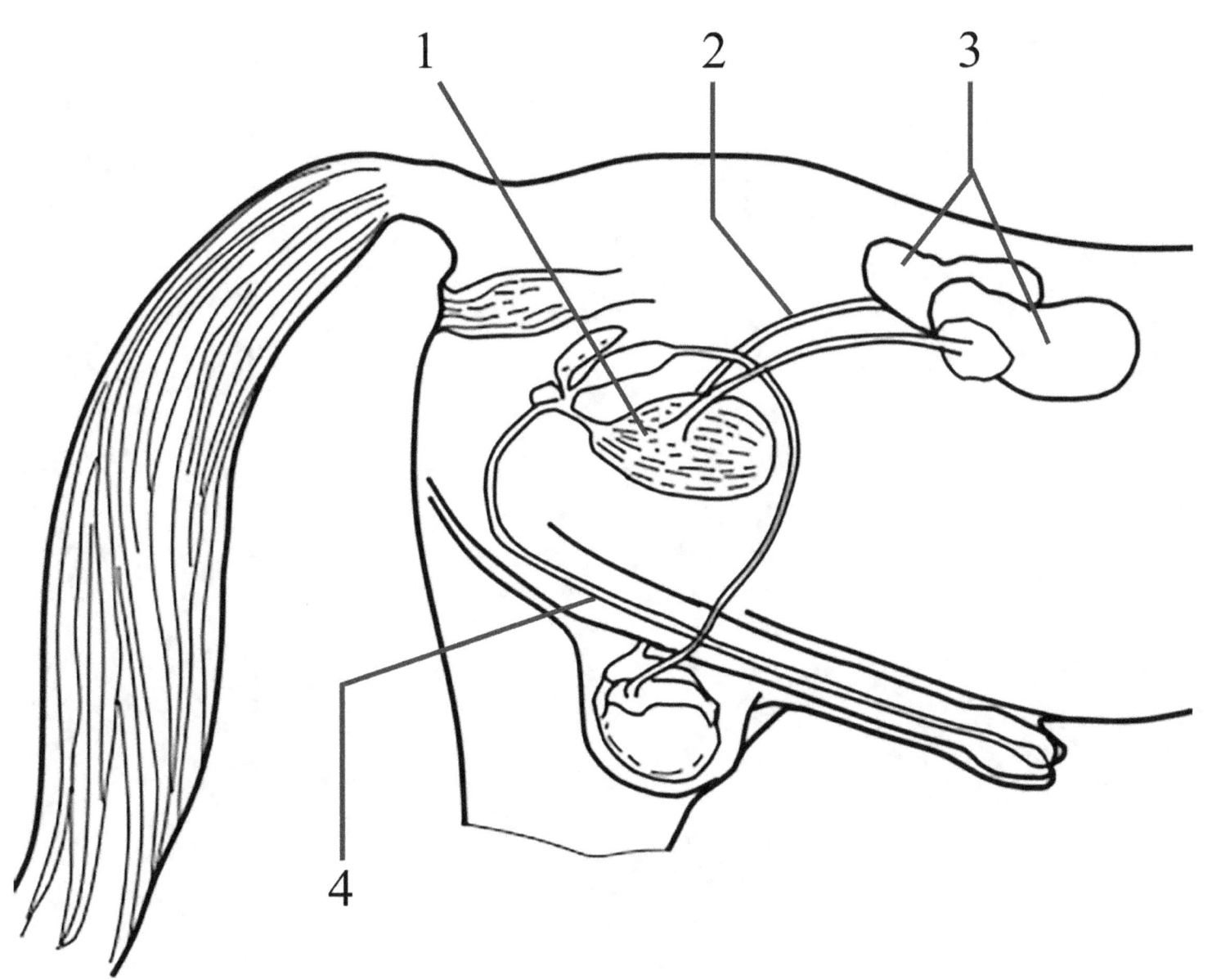

MARE URINARY SYSTEM

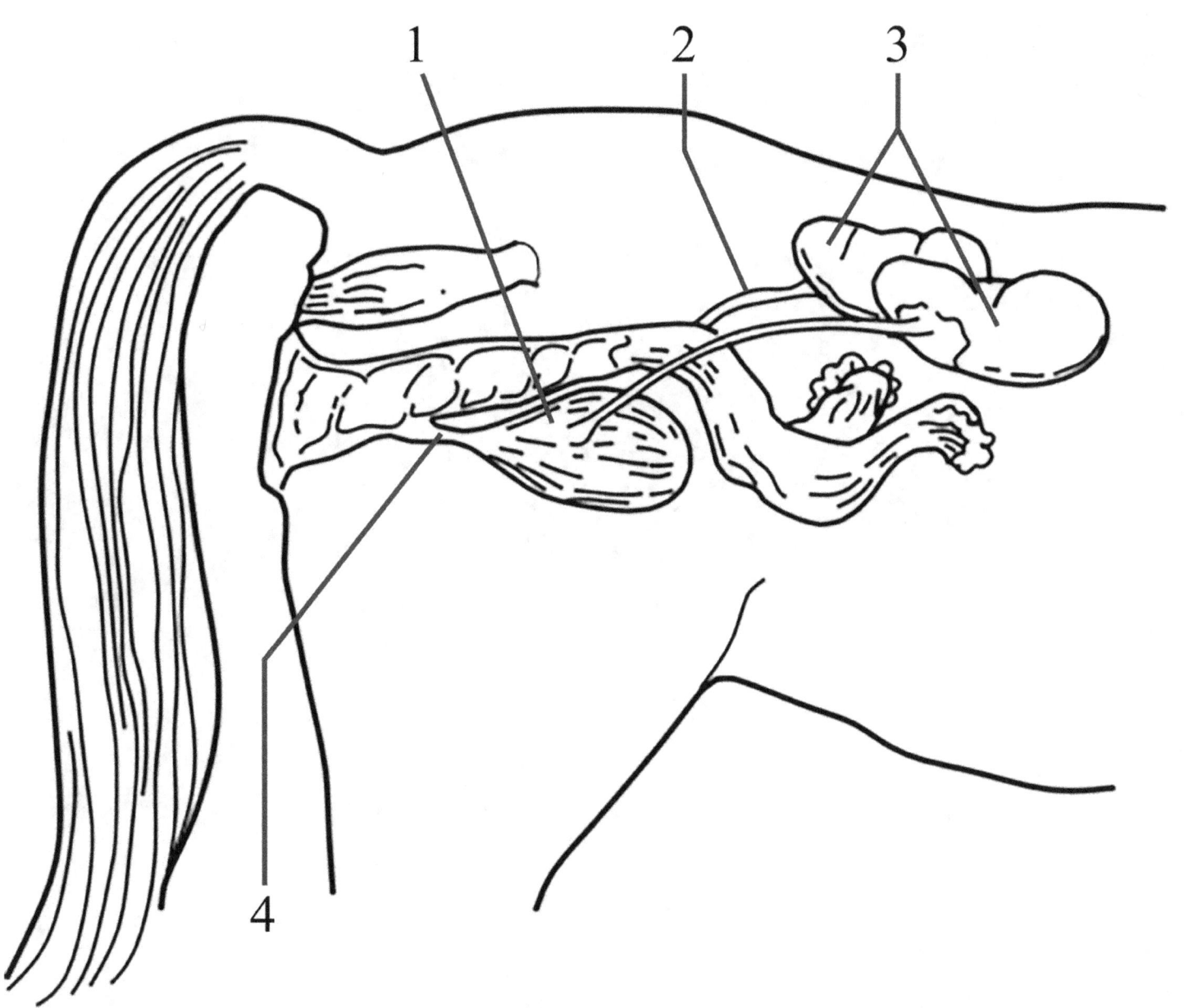

EXTERIOR VIEW OF STALLION REPRODUCTIVE ORGAN

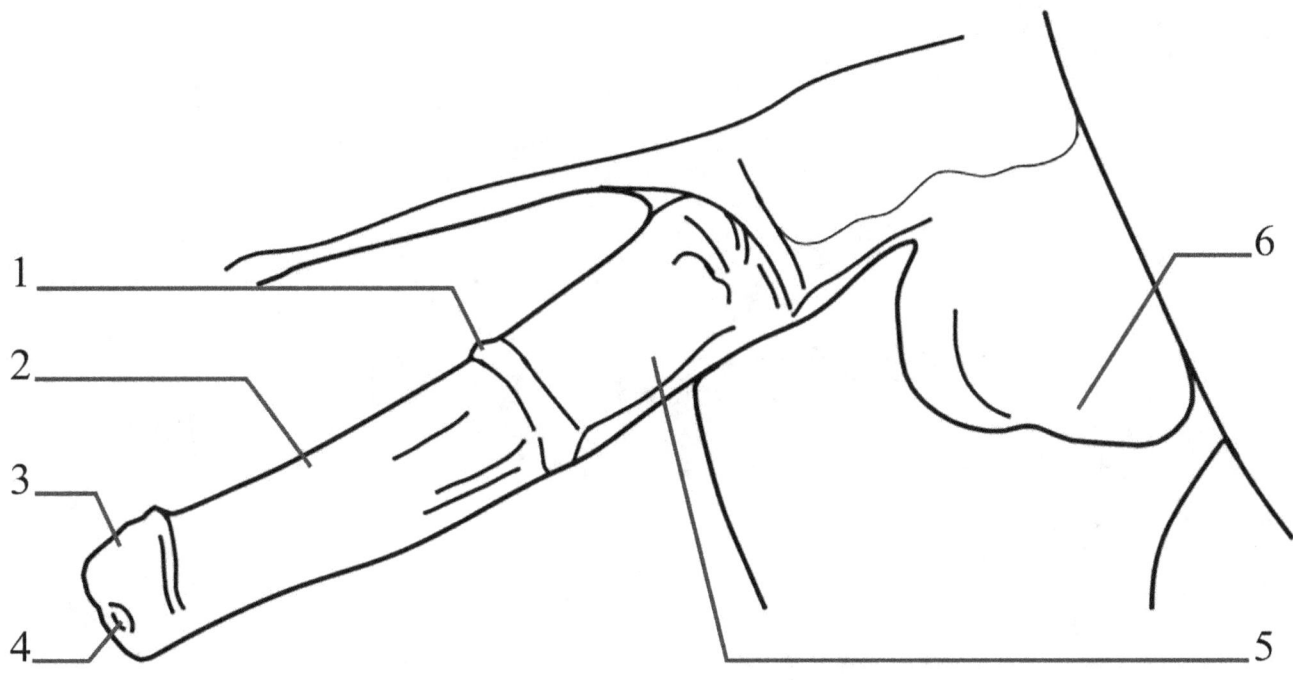

STALLION REPRODUCTIVE TRACT

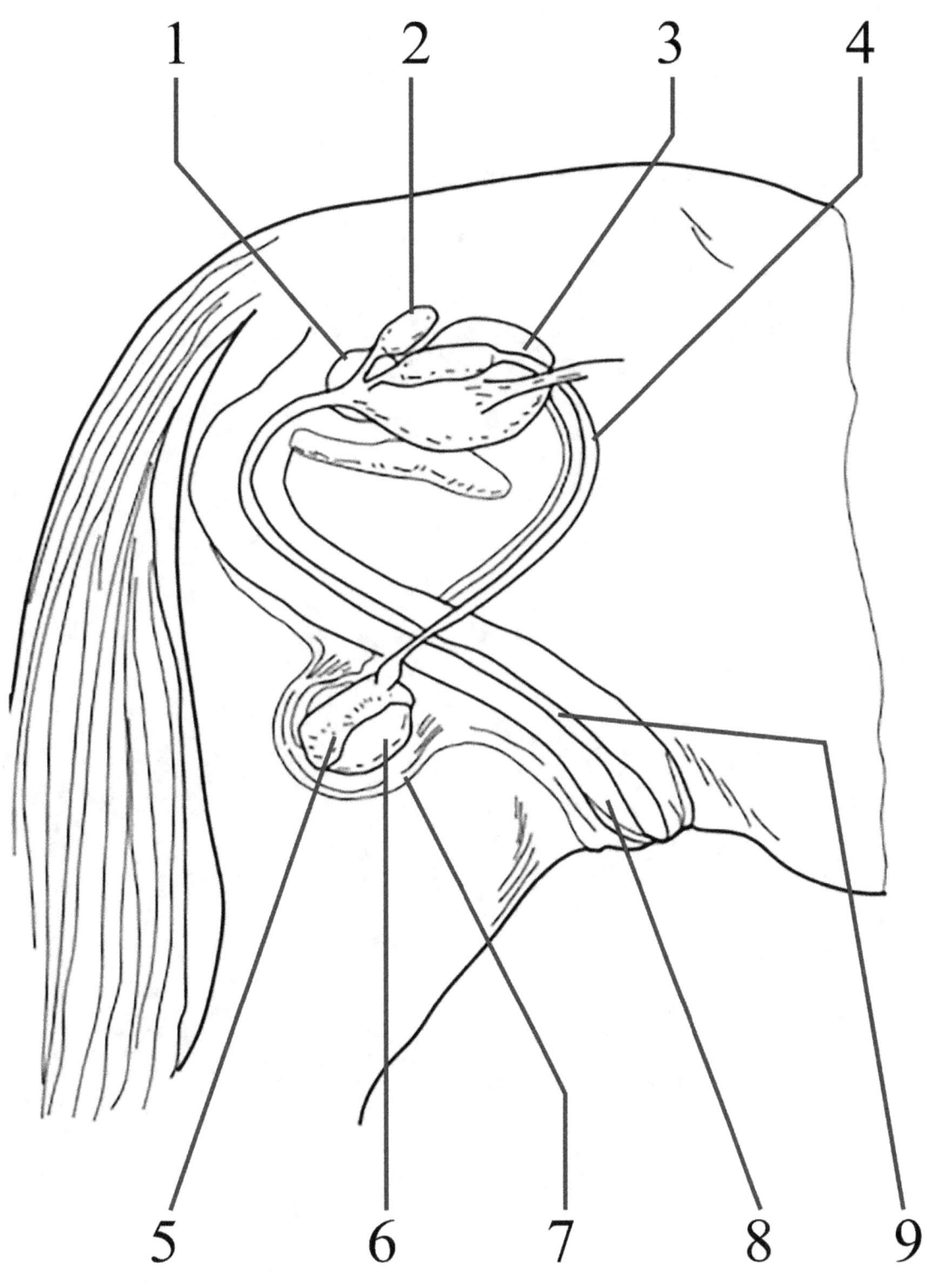

MARE GENITAL TRACT

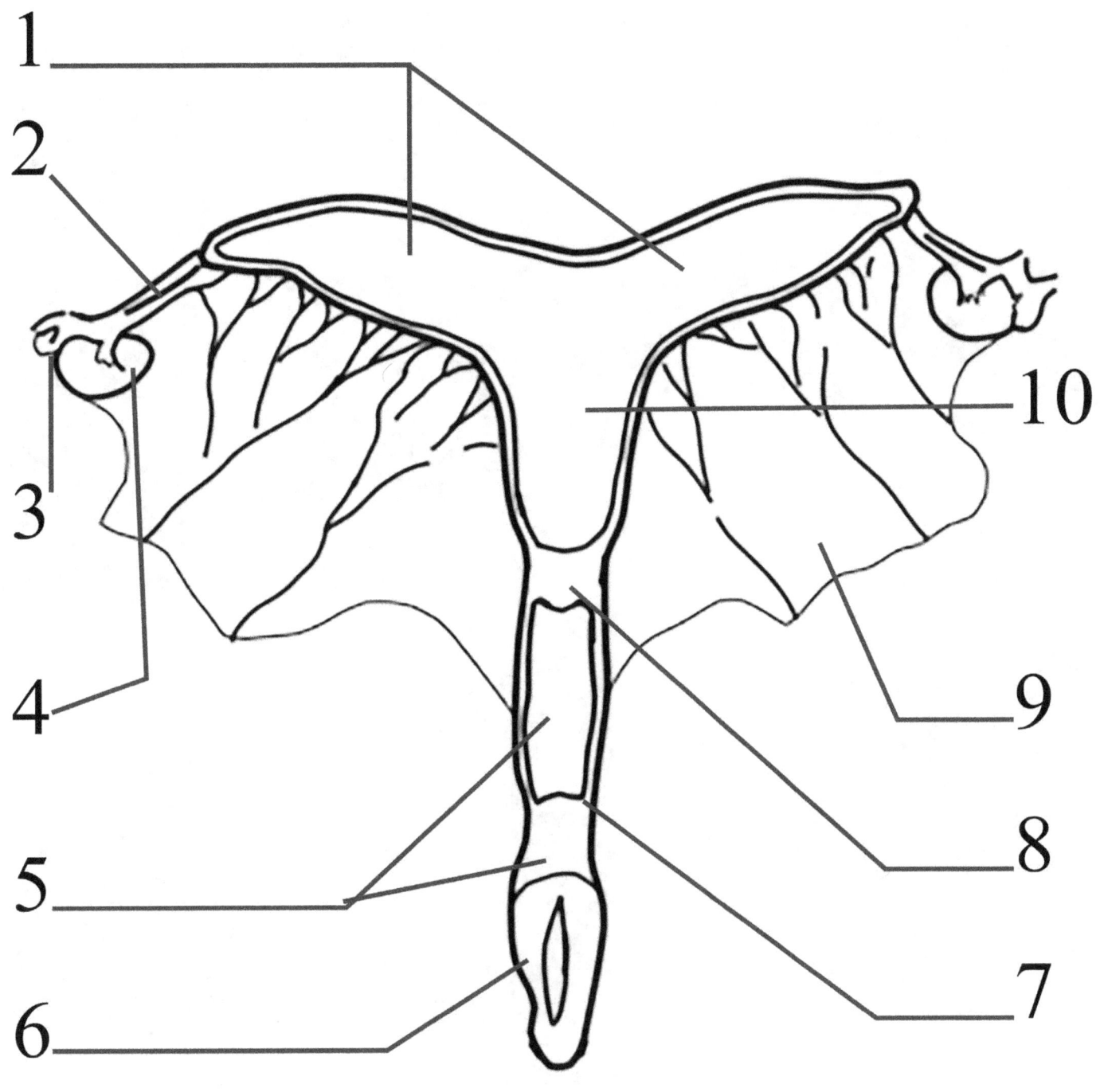

MARE REPRODUCTIVE TRACT

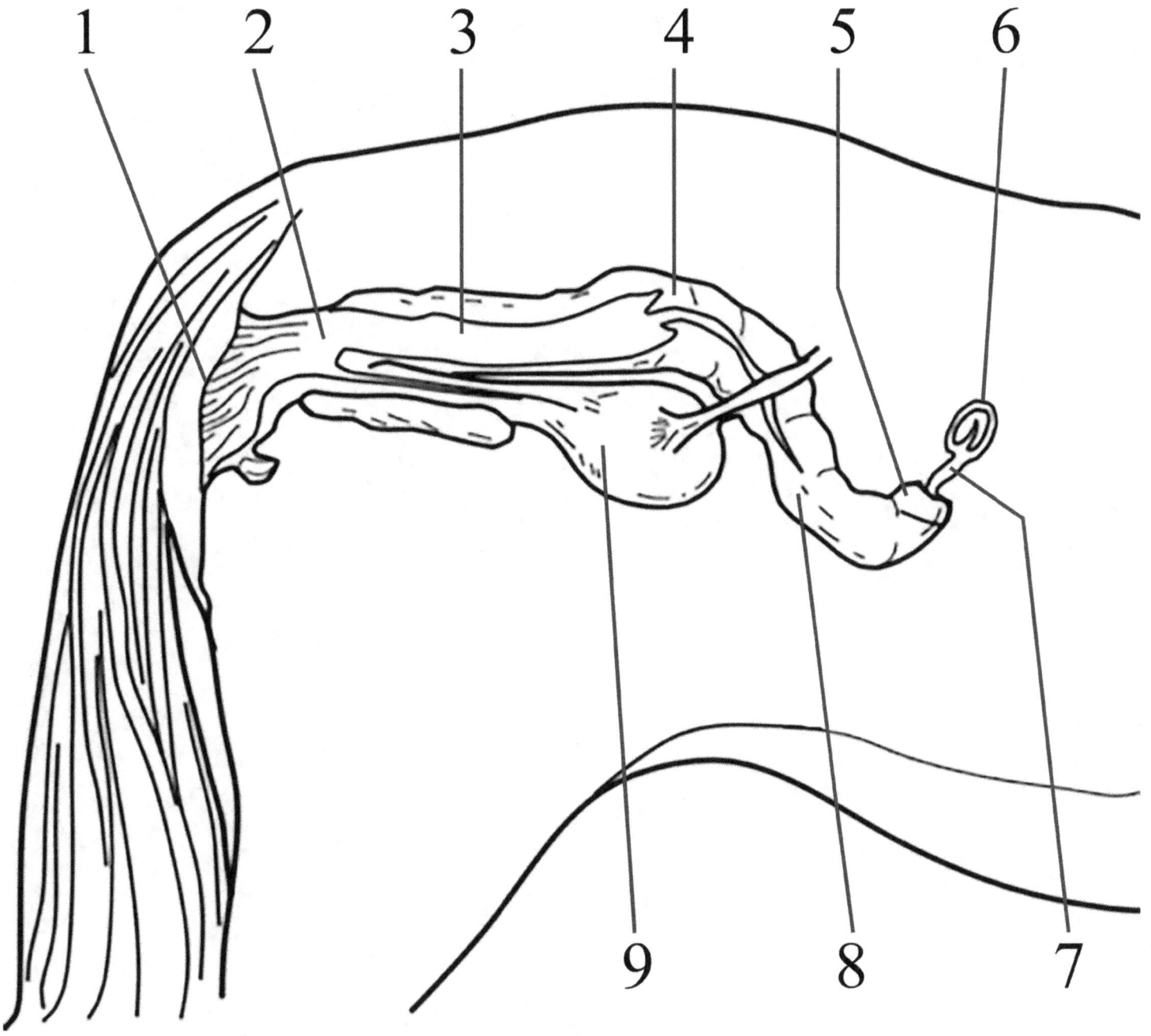

EXTERNAL ANATOMY OF HORSE

COMPLETE SKELETON OF A HORSE

1. Jaw
2. Bars
3. Skull
4. Atlas
5. Axis
6. Neck vertebrae
7. Scapula
8. Lumbar vertebrae
9. Point of hip
10. Lumbosacral joint
11. Sacrum
12. Pelvis
13. Hip joint
14. Femur
15. Tibia
16. Hock
17. Cannon
18. Splint bone
19. Patella
20. Rib cage
21. Sternum
22. Pisiform bone
23. Sesamoid bone
24. Navicular bone
25. Pedal bone
26. Short pastern bone
27. Long pastern bone
28. Knee
29. Radius
30. Elbow joint
31. Humerus
32. Point of shoulder

FORELIMB

1. Scapula
2. Radius
3. Cannon
4. Proximal or first phalanx
5. Middle or second phalanx
6. Distal or third phalanx
7. Coffin joint
8. Pastern joint
9. Fetlock joint
10. Splint bone
11. Accessory carpal bone
12. Elbow joint
13. Humerus
14. Shoulder joint

ANTERIOR VIEW OF EQUINE CARPUS

1. Radius bone
2. Intermediate carpal bone
3. Ulnar carpal bone
4. Fourth carpal bone
5. Fourth metacarpal bone
6. Third metacarpal bone
7. Second metacarpal bone
8. Second carpal bone
9. Third carpal bone
10. Radial carpal bone

HIND LIMB

1. Ilium
2. Hip joint
3. Femur
4. Patella
5. Tibia
6. Cannon
7. Fetlock joint
8. Proximal or first phalanx
9. Distal or third phalanx
10. Coffin joint
11. Middle or second phalanx
12. Pastern joint
13. Splint bone
14. Hock joint
15. Tuber calcanei
16. Stifle joint
17. Ischiatic tuberosity

EQUINE TARSUS AND STIFLE

1. Tibia
2. Talus
3. Central tarsal bone
4. Third tarsal bone
5. Third metatarsal
6. Fused first and second tarsal bones
7. Fourth tarsal bone
8. Calcaneus

SPINAL CORD OF A YOUNG HORSE

1. Cervical part
2. Thoracic part
3. Lumbar part
4. Sacral part
5. Lumbosacral foramen
6. Lumbar thickening
7. Conus medullaris and cauda equina
8. Cervical thickening
9. Intervertebral foramen
10. Lateral vertebral foramen
11. Medulla oblongata and cervical part

HORSE SKULL

1. Canine tooth
2. Premolar 1 (wolf's tooth)
3. Maxillary cheek teeth
4. Bony orbit
5. Temporomandibular joint
6. Incisor teeth
7. Mandibular cheek teeth
8. Mandible

EQUINE DENTISTRY

1. Molar
2. Premolar
3. Premolar 1 (wolf's tooth)
4. Canine
5. Incisor

HORSE HOOF

1. Cannon bone
2. Fetlock joint
3. Skin
4. Long pastern bone (first phalanx)
5. Pastern joint
6. Second phalanx
7. Hoof wall
8. Sole
9. Coffin bone
10. Frog
11. Digital cushion
12. Bulb of heel
13. Navicular bone
14. Coffin joint
15. Sigmoidal bone

EXTERIOR VIEW AND GROUND SURFACE OF THE HOOF

1. Toe
2. Stratum medium of the hoof wall
3. White line
4. Apex of frog
5. Bar
6. Angle of bar
7. Angle of wall
8. Cleft of frog
9. Heel
10. Bulb of heel
11. Lateral sulcus
12. Sole
13. Coronary band
14. Wall of the hoof

LIMB TENDON AND LIGAMENT

1. Carpus
2. Cannon bone
3. Inferior check ligament
4. Exterior branch of the suspensory ligament
5. Superficial digital flexor tendon
6. Sesamoid bones
7. Body of suspensory ligament
8. Accessory carpal bone
9. Splint bone
10. Deep digital flexor tendon
11. Superficial digital flexor tendon
12. Branches of the suspensory ligament
13. Sesamoid ligaments

DORSAL VIEW OF HORSE BRAIN WITH SECTIONED LEFT HEMISPHERE

1. Olfactory bulb
2. Cerebral cortex
3. Head of caudate nucleus
4. Choroid plexus of lateral vertebrae
5. Septum pellucidum
6. Ammon's horn (pes hippocampi)
7. Accessory nerve
8. Vermis
9. Cerebellar hemisphere
10. Gyri
11. Sulci
12. Cerebral hemisphere
13. Longitudinal cerebral tissue

EQUINE EYE

1. Conjunctiva
2. Ciliary body
3. Eyelid
4. Aqueous humor
5. Cornea
6. Pupil
7. Anterior chamber
8. Iris
9. Eyelid
10. Third eyelid
11. Optic nerve
12. Vitreous chamber
13. Sclera
14. Choroid
15. Retina
16. Lacrimal gland
17. Anterior segment
18. Posterior segment

EXTERIOR VIEW OF EQUINE EYE

1. Third eyelid
2. Lacrimal puncta
3. Lacrimal caruncle
4. Openings of tarsal glands
5. Lens (visible through the pupil)
6. Iris
7. Sclera
8. Lacrimal gland
9. Corpora nigra

ANATOMY OF A HORSE TONGUE

1. Apex of tongue
2. Lingual frenulum
3. Sublingual caruncle
4. Fungiform papillae
5. Filiform papillae
6. Body of tongue
7. Foliate papillae
8. Stump of palatoglossal
9. Vallate papillae
10. Median laryngeal recess
11. Corniculate process of arytenoid cartilage
12. Glottic
13. Laryngeal ventricle
14. Epiglottis
15. Palatine tonsil
16. Lingual tonsil
17. Root of tongue

EQUINE EAR

1. Pinna
2. Ear canal
3. Eardrum
4. Tympanic cavity
5. Eustachian tube opening
6. Auditory nerve
7. Cochlea
8. Ossicles (hammer, anvil, and stirrup)
9. Vestibular system

STRUCTURE OF HORSE SKIN

1. Hair shaft
2. Sebaceous gland
3. Epidermis
4. Dermis
5. Subcutaneous layer
6. Hair follicle
7. Sweat gland

EQUINE RESPIRATORY SYSTEM

1. Guttural pouch
2. Nasal cavity
3. Nostrils
4. Bronchus
5. Pharynx
6. Larynx
7. Trachea
8. Lung
9. Bronchioles
10. Alveoli

VENTRAL VIEW OF THE LUNGS

1. Cardiac notch
2. Deep cervical vessels
3. Right lung
4. Accessory lobe
5. Lobar bronchus
6. Cranial lobes
7. Pulmonary veins
8. Left lung
9. Oesophagus
10. Caudal lobes

DORSAL VIEW OF BRONCHIAL TREE

1. Lobar bronchus
2. Left tracheobronchial lymph nodes
3. Principal bronchus
4. Lobar bronchus
5. Segmental bronchus
6. Pulmonary lymph nodes
7. Middle tracheobronchial lymph nodes
8. Tracheal bifurcation
9. Right tracheobronchial lymph nodes

DIGESTIVE SYSTEM OF A HORSE

1. Oesophagus
2. Stomach
3. Small Intestine
4. Colon
5. Rectum
6. Cecum

THE EQUINE STOMACH

1. Saccus caecus - non-glandular system
2. Margo plicatus
3. Fundic gland region
4. Glandular section
5. Pyloric gland section
6. Pylorus
7. Start of duodenum - small intestine
8. Oesophagus
9. Cardiac sphincter valve

LARGE INTESTINE OF A HORSE

1. Cecum
2. Large intestine
3. Pelvic Flexure
4. Rectum

EQUINE HEART

1. Left atrium
2. Pulmonary veins
3. Coronary groove
4. Aorta
5. Pulmonary trunk
6. Brachiocephalic trunk
7. Cranial vena cava
8. Right atrium
9. Right ventricle
10. Interventricular groove
11. Left ventricle
12. Aorta valve
13. Pectinate muscle
14. Coronary vessels
15. Interventricular septum
16. Chordae tendineae

STALLION URINARY SYSTEM

1. Bladder
2. Ureter
3. Kidneys
4. Urethra

MARE URINARY SYSTEM

1. Bladder
2. Ureter
3. Kidneys
4. Urethra

EXTERIOR VIEW OF STALLION REPRODUCTIVE ORGAN

1. Preputial Ring
2. Free Body of Penis
3. Glans Penis
4. Urethral Process
5. Inner Lamina of Prepuce
6. Scrotum containing Testes

STALLION REPRODUCTIVE TRACT ANATOMY

1. Prostate gland
2. Vesicular gland
3. Bladder
4. Vas deferens
5. Epididymis
6. Testicle
7. Scrotum
8. Glans penis
9. Urethra

MARE GENITAL TRACT

1. Uterine horns
2. Oviduct
3. Infundibulum
4. Ovary
5. Vagina
6. Vulva
7. Transverse fold
8. Cervix
9. Broad ligament
10. Uterine body

MARE REPRODUCTIVE TRACT

1. Vulva
2. Vestibule
3. Vagina
4. Cervix
5. Horn of uterus
6. Ovary
7. Fallopian tube
8. Body of uterus
9. Bladder

EXTERNAL ANATOMY OF HORSE

1. Forelock
2. Facial crest
3. Muzzle
4. Chin groove
5. Throat
6. Jugular groove
7. Shoulder
8. Forearm
9. Knee
10. Fore cannon
11. Pastern
12. Belly
13. Stifle
14. Hind cannon
15. Coronet
16. Wall of hoof
17. Heel
18. Fetlock
19. Point of hock
20. Gaskin
21. Tail
22. Thigh
23. Buttock
24. Hip
25. Flank
26. Dock
27. Hindquarter
28. Croup
29. Loins
30. Back
31. Withers
32. Neck
33. Mane
34. Crest
35. Poll

www.ingramcontent.com/pod-product-compliance
Lightning Source LLC
Chambersburg PA
CBHW081534220526
45467CB00010B/3190